Undefeated

Navigating Chronic Fatigue and Fibromyalgia to Wellness

By
Well-Being Publishing

To You,

Thank you!

Table of Contents

Introduction:
The Journey to Wellness Begins

Embarking on a journey to wellness can be both daunting and hopeful. When the invisible weight of chronic fatigue syndrome (CFS) and fibromyalgia (FM) rests on your shoulders, it can feel like you're wading through fog—both misunderstood and misdiagnosed too often. But here, within these pages, lies a map through that fog, a guide crafted with empathy and expertise to lead you toward understanding and managing these complex conditions. It's a path lit with practical advice, not just to live with CFS and FM, but to thrive despite them. Together, we'll explore the intricacies of your symptoms, the insights from the latest research, and the personal stories of those who've walked this path before you. This book isn't just a collection of information; it's a beacon of hope, a source of strength, and a community of shared experiences. Let's take this first step into your journey to wellness with courage, knowing that with every page turned, you're moving closer to a life you'll author, one of resilience, health, and peace.

Chapter 1:
Understanding Chronic Fatigue Syndrome (CFS) and Fibromyalgia (FM)

Embarking on the journey to wellness, it's vital to lay a solid foundation with an understanding of Chronic Fatigue Syndrome (CFS) and Fibromyalgia (FM)—conditions that are as enigmatic as they are debilitating. CFS, with its core hallmark of persistent and unexplained fatigue, can feel like an anchor, weighing on every aspect of your day. Life with FM is often marred by widespread pain, akin to a symphony of discomfort playing throughout your body, with tender points that react with a sharpness that startles and drains. Both conditions are notorious for their ability to masquerade as other ailments, making diagnosis a challenge that requires not just a doctor's insight but your own attunement to your body's distress signals. Because they so frequently walk hand in hand, CFS and FM share a common thread, weaving through your daily life, creating overlapping challenges that make each day unpredictable. But within the tapestry of symptoms there lies a pattern, and once decoded, it becomes possible to face these challenges with a measure of grace and determination. This chapter isn't just about dissecting symptoms; it's about grasping the complexity of your experiences, recognizing your struggles, and affirming that they're more than mere entries in medical charts—they're the whispers of your body's needs, begging to be heard, acknowledged, and addressed.

The Symptoms and Diagnostic Criteria

Embarking on the exploration of Chronic Fatigue Syndrome (CFS) and Fibromyalgia (FM) means first understanding the complex array of symptoms that sufferers navigate daily. Often, the journey to a diagnosis is a labyrinth of consultations, tests, and self-reflection. It is a path marked by uncertainty, but clarity begins with recognition of the patterns that define these conditions.

CFS is characterized primarily by persistent and overwhelming fatigue that isn't alleviated by rest. This fatigue often hampers daily activities, going beyond typical tiredness. Sufferers might find themselves unable to maintain their normal work or social life, a stark change from their pre-illness activity levels.

Common to both CFS and FM is the presence of pain—an uninvited guest that persists and migrates with little to no apparent cause. FM is particularly known for chronic widespread pain across the musculoskeletal system, presenting as a constant dull ache. Accompanying this pain one often finds tender points—specific areas that hurt when pressure is applied—though these are not exclusively indicative of FM.

However, pain and fatigue do not sail alone. They're accompanied by a fleet of symptoms like sleep disturbances where sufferers may wake up feeling just as exhausted as when they lay down. CFS and FM can both disrupt the restorative stages of sleep, leaving one feeling weary and unrefreshed.

Cognitive difficulties, often informally referred to as "brain fog," can make concentration and memory a daunting challenge. Simple tasks and decisions might suddenly feel like monumental undertakings. It's as if layers of gauze wrap around one's thoughts, making every intellectual attempt a bit more strenuous.

For a diagnosis of CFS, criteria established by medical entities, such as the Centers for Disease Control and Prevention, are often referred to. They dictate that in addition to debilitating fatigue, one must experience a subset of additional symptoms, including sore throat, lymph node pain, muscle ache, multi-joint pain, headaches, and a prolonged worsening of symptoms post-exertion, often described as "post-exertional malaise."

FM's diagnosis, on the other hand, takes into account the widespread pain index (WPI) and the symptom severity scale (SS). A higher count in these measures, together with the history of symptoms over a three-month period, contributes to a FM diagnosis. Unlike CFS, there is a stronger emphasis on the number and severity of tender points with FM.

It's crucial to remember that CFS and FM are exclusionary diagnoses. This means that these diagnoses are often only confirmed after other possible conditions have been ruled out. Hence, a thorough medical evaluation for each person is crucial, considering that symptoms can mimic or coincide with other illnesses.

Often overlooked, but vitally important, are the emotional repercussions of CFS and FM. It's not unusual for those affected to experience depression or anxiety, both as a reaction to chronic pain and fatigue and as intertwined symptoms of their conditions. This emotional toll underscores the need for a multidimensional approach to diagnosis and management.

It's worth noting that these conditions don't have a one-size-fits-all presentation. Symptoms can range from mild to severe, and might fluctuate over time. Some days are better, and some are markedly worse—a pattern that can be frustrating and disheartening.

In recent years, the diagnostic process has become somewhat more streamlined, with the development of diagnostic criteria more sensitive to the typical presentation of symptoms. These criteria are foundational, providing medical professionals with a guideline, yet each person's narrative holds the key to personalizing their diagnosis and subsequent management.

Furthermore, with such a wide spectrum of symptoms, CFS and FM often coexist with other conditions, such as irritable bowel syndrome, interstitial cystitis, migraines, and various autoimmune disorders. Identifying and managing these comorbid conditions is a critical aspect of overall treatment strategy.

Understanding symptoms and the road to diagnosis is a significant step toward empowerment. Knowledge of these disorders arms those affected with the vocabulary to articulate their experiences to healthcare providers and loved ones. It's a pivotal component of the compass that navigates the complex terrain of chronic illness management.

The symptoms of CFS and FM are not just disruptive; they are often invisible to outsiders, making validation and understanding from others sometimes elusive. Thus, the diagnostic criteria serve as a necessary bridge between subjective experience and objective assessment—clarifying a path for therapy and support.

Equipped with an understanding of these symptoms and diagnostic benchmarks, we succinctly pave a way for better communication, targeted research, and comprehensive care, all to Foster a future where individuals with CFS and FM can reclaim their vitality and well-being.

The Overlapping Challenges of CFS and FM

For anyone faced with the complexities of Chronic Fatigue Syndrome (CFS) and Fibromyalgia (FM), understanding the overlapping challenges these conditions bring is crucial. These syndromes share a myriad of symptoms and can often co-occur, complicating diagnosis and management. But despite the challenges, there are strategies and hope for those affected.

At the heart of both conditions is a profound, persistent fatigue that's not alleviated by rest. This isn't the tiredness you feel after a long day; it's a deep-seated exhaustion that can make the simplest activity seem like climbing a mountain. Beyond that, pain is prevalent in FM and can also be a component of CFS, manifesting in a generalized, widespread fashion that can sometimes be debilitating.

Understanding the symptoms is just the starting point. The real challenge lies in the fact that both conditions can feature 'flares', periods of heightened symptoms that can throw off your routines and require a sudden need to scale back activities. Flares are unpredictable, which means planning becomes a tentative activity, and patients often feel they are at the mercy of their conditions.

Cognitive difficulties—often referred to as "brain fog"—are also a common shared trait. As if wading through a mental marsh, individuals may struggle with focus, memory, and clarity of thought. This aspect can be particularly distressing, as it affects personal and professional life and one's sense of identity and capability.

Both syndromes are also characterized by disrupted sleep. You might think that being so fatigued would mean sleep comes easily, but that's far from the case. Rest can be elusive, and when it comes, it's often unrefreshing. Poor sleep exacerbates other symptoms, forming a relentless cycle that's hard to break.

Mood disturbances also intertwine with CFS and FM. Dealing with chronic pain and fatigue can take a toll on anyone's emotional wellbeing, leading to anxiety and depression. The invisible nature of these conditions can lead to a lack of understanding from others, adding an additional emotional burden.

Physical symptoms like irritable bowel syndrome, headaches, and sensitivity to stimuli are other arenas where the challenges of CFS and FM overlap. It's not just the pain or fatigue that one has to manage, but a whole host of body systems that seem to rebel simultaneously.

Diagnostic challenges lie in the symptom overlap between CFS and FM, which often leads to a circuitous path in search of answers. Since there's no definitive test, a diagnosis is typically a process of exclusion, and the overlap can cloud the clinical picture, making it harder for practitioners to pin down a precise diagnosis.

Treatment is another area of conflation. With no known cure, approaches focus on symptom management. Yet, because of the symptom overlap, patients may find themselves on a medication regimen for CFS, only to realize that some interventions align more closely with FM treatment protocols. Consequently, treatment often requires a trial-and-error approach to find what works best for the individual.

Stigma and misunderstanding can be just as debilitating as the symptoms themselves. Because both CFS and FM can be elusive to those who've never experienced them, sufferers can face skepticism from acquaintances and even healthcare professionals. Advocating for oneself becomes a necessary, yet exhausting, part of the journey.

Navigating daily life when your resources are so limited is difficult. Pacing becomes a way of life, listening intently to your body's signals for rest. Strategies for managing energy levels are vital, involving a delicate balance of rest and activity, and there's a constant need to adapt as symptoms fluctuate.

Despite these challenges, it is within the interstices of uncertainty and struggle where resilience can bloom. Patients find strength they never knew they had, develop communities of support through shared experience, and often emerge with a changed, but in many ways richer, outlook on life.

It's important to remember you're not alone. Many face these challenges. Yet, within the overlap of CFS and FM, there also lies a community, a group of individuals who understand what it means to persist through fatigue and pain. Here, mutual understanding serves as a foundation for shared learning and support.

The key to living with these overlapping challenges is to manage the conditions, not to let them manage you. This means being proactive about treatment options, creative in coping strategies, and compassionate with yourself. A multi-disciplinary approach that includes medication, diet, exercise, therapy, and a strong support network proves to be the most beneficial.

In essence, the story of CFS and FM is one of perseverance, of acknowledging the limitations and finding the courage to push through them. It's a narrative punctuated by good days and bad, but also by hope and the relentless pursuit of wellness. While the path may be winding, the strength found in journeying it is immeasurable.

Chapter 2:
The History and Science Behind CFS and FM

As we delve deeper into the enigma of Chronic Fatigue Syndrome (CFS) and Fibromyalgia (FM), it's imperative to explore the rich tapestry of their history and the ever-evolving landscape of science that seeks to decode their mysteries. These conditions aren't just modern-day afflictions; their presence has been hinted at through medical literature for centuries, although they've often been misunderstood and wrongly dismissed. In this chapter, we'll trace the path blazed by intrepid researchers and patients alike, examining breakthroughs that have shed light on the biological complexities inherent to CFS and FM. While the journey has been arduous, with each scientific endeavor, from gene mapping to the study of neuroinflammation, we edge closer to unraveling the intricate web of factors driving these disorders. Understanding the groundwork laid by history and science is more than an academic pursuit—it's a beacon of hope illuminating the way forward for countless individuals striving toward wellness in a world that's just beginning to grasp the far-reaching impact of these conditions.

Tracing the Origins: A Historical Perspective

The story of Chronic Fatigue Syndrome (CFS) and Fibromyalgia (FM) is one that's as perplexing as the conditions themselves. While the medical community today debates various aspects of these syndromes, the puzzle actually dates back several centuries. Understanding where we've come from can shed some light on where we stand with CFS and FM now—and where we're heading.

Historically, we can trace symptoms akin to those of CFS and FM to the 18th century with descriptions revolving around 'muscle rheumatism' and 'neurasthenia', the latter term coined by neurologist George Miller Beard in 1869. This was a time when the medical world was just beginning to appreciate the interconnectedness of the body and mind, and these terms were used loosely to describe a plethora of symptoms that ranged from fatigue to depression to musculoskeletal pain.

As time marched on, these syndromes took on various names and faces, often colored by the prevailing medical theories of the eras. The concept of 'fibrositis', introduced in the early 20th century, implicated inflammation of the muscle's connective tissue as the cause of pain—a theory we know today to be inaccurate regarding FM. Due to the lack of clear-cut diagnostic markers, these conditions often resided on the fringes of medical legitimacy, leading to immense patient frustration.

The plight of CFS surfaced more prominently in the medical literature in the mid to late 20th century, particularly following a cluster of cases in the 1980s at Lake Tahoe, Nevada, that seemed epidemic in nature, bringing about the term 'Chronic Epstein-Barr Virus Syndrome'. The event was a turning point, as it highlighted the complexity and the critical need for research into CFS.

The evolution of FM took a similar path. It wasn't until 1990 that the American College of Rheumatology established the first diagnostic criteria for FM, primarily focusing on the characteristic tender points and widespread pain that patients experience. It was a watershed moment—patients finally had something concrete to associate with their suffering, and physicians had a guideline to diagnosis.

Yet, despite these strides in recognition, understanding the root causes of CFS and FM has been equal parts challenging and contentious. Theories have oscillated between viral origins, immune system dysfunctions, hormonal disparities, and even psychological causations. This has led to a fragmentation of perspectives both within and outside the medical field, often leaving patients caught in the crossfire of debates and disbelief.

However, amidst the debates, the patient voices have consistently echoed a need for validation and effective management strategies. Advocacy groups emerged, patient-led research became more prevalent, and a push toward bio-psycho-social models of disease gained traction. These efforts have been crucial in navigating the maze of symptoms and treatment options.

Scientific curiosity has also been piqued by the discovery of the potential role of the central nervous system and the concept of central sensitization in both CFS and FM. The realization that the brain could be magnifying pain signals or misinterpreting energy production and usage provided fresh angles for treatment and research. This mind-body connection concept has been gradually making its way into mainstream treatment protocols, offering a glimmer of hope for those affected.

Alongside these scientific discoveries, remarkable stories have unfolded—stories of remarkable resilience, relentless pursuits of wellness, and community building. These narratives contribute to the tapestry of CFS and FM history, adding depth and strength to the push for progress and understanding.

In the contemporary era, medical technology and research modalities have provided tools previously unavailable to early investigators of these conditions—tools like functional MRI to examine brain activity, advanced blood tests for biomarkers of inflammation, and genetic assays to probe predispositions to these illnesses. Each offers a potential piece to the ever-expanding puzzle.

It's worth acknowledging that as much as CFS and FM are about history, they're also about individuals. Each person coping with these conditions carries on a legacy of those who have struggled, advocated, and forged paths in the face of obscurity and skepticism. There's an innate strength found in the knowledge that one is a part of something larger—a narrative of endurance and determination.

With breakthroughs in the realms of treatment and a growing awareness in both the medical field and public consciousness, the future for CFS and FM holds promise. It's about building on the past, learning from mistakes, celebrating victories no matter how small, and above all, maintaining an indefatigable spirit of inquiry that holds patient wellbeing as its core.

In the following chapters, we will delve deeper into the biological underpinnings and the latest research that shines light on these mysterious conditions. But for now, appreciating the long journey of CFS and FM is essential. It's a reminder that even amidst chronic illness, there is a rich heritage that sees sufferers not as mere patients, but as pioneers in a story that continues to unfold.

And so, we stand on the shoulders of the many—doctors, researchers, patients, and advocates—whose dedicated pursuit of knowledge and wellness has led us here. As you embark on your journey towards managing CFS and FM, the past offers the strongest foundation, and history can serve as the greatest teacher. Let's carry that legacy forward with optimism and determination for a brighter, healthier future ahead.

The Biological Underpinnings and Latest Research

As we delve deeper into understanding Chronic Fatigue Syndrome (CFS) and Fibromyalgia (FM), it's essential to unravel the biological mysteries that have confounded experts for decades. Recent advancements in research shine a light on the multifaceted nature of these conditions, helping us piece together a more coherent narrative of their origins and pathological processes.

At the forefront of this quest are scientists exploring the intricate dance of the human immune system. It's now becoming clear that both CFS and FM may involve a dysregulated immune response. People with these conditions often report a viral or bacterial infection preceding their symptoms, prompting researchers to consider that an ongoing, abnormal immune reaction to an initial trigger may be sustaining the illness.

Issues related to energy metabolism also show promise in revealing secrets of these conditions. Mitochondria, the energy powerhouses of the cells, may not function optimally in patients with CFS and FM, resulting in reduced energy output and persistent fatigue. Studies are investigating not just the functionality of these mitochondria but also the nutrients and co-factors that support their health.

While the immune system and energy production are significant pieces of this puzzle, a cascade of hormonal disturbances is also involved. The hypothalamus-pituitary-adrenal (HPA) axis, a central hormone production pathway, often appears disrupted in those with CFS and FM. This disruption can affect everything from sleep cycles to pain perception, offering a potential explanation for the broad array of symptoms experienced.

The role of the central nervous system (CNS) should not be understated either. Research indicates heightened CNS sensitivity in CFS and FM patients, leading to an exaggerated pain response to stimuli that wouldn't cause discomfort in healthy individuals—a phenomenon known as central sensitization. This may help to elucidate the relentless pain that characterizes fibromyalgia in particular.

Advancements in genetics offer another fruitful avenue, as scientists look for hereditary patterns that might predispose someone to these conditions. While no single "CFS gene" or "FM gene" has been identified, genetic research may uncover a predisposition that could interact with environmental factors to trigger the diseases. Understanding these genetic factors can lead to personalized approaches in management and treatment.

Infections continue to attract attention, with some studies suggesting that certain microbes might act as catalysts for the development of CFS and FM. The theory here is that microbes may prompt a change in the body's immune response, or directly affect muscle and nerve functions, contributing to the symptoms of fibromyalgia and chronic fatigue syndrome.

The link to the gut-brain axis is another compelling chapter of contemporary research. The gut microbiome and its role in systemic health vastly impacts conditions like CFS and FM. Imbalance in gut flora—dysbiosis—has been associated with the severity of symptoms, drawing researchers to probe into the benefits of dietary changes and probiotic interventions.

Moving beyond single-factor theories, the modern approach appreciates the complexity and interplay of various systems in the body. This bio-psycho-social model acknowledges that emotional stressors can have tangible biological effects and vice versa. It's a nuanced perspective that aligns with the variable nature of CFS and FM, recognizing that multiple triggers and ongoing stressors may intertwine to sustain the illness.

On the horizon, there's a burgeoning interest in the potential of precision medicine. This cutting-edge field aims to tailor treatment plans to an individual's unique biological makeup, including their genomic profile, lifestyle, and environmental exposures. For those living with CFS and FM, this could mean a future of highly personalized care designed to address their specific needs.

The envelope theory has also garnered attention as a metaphor for the energy limitations characteristic of CFS and FM. By conceiving of energy as a finite resource—much like the space in an envelope—patients and healthcare providers can visualize the need to budget activities to prevent overshooting one's energy limits and causing post-exertional malaise.

An understudied but potentially significant factor in CFS and FM is the role of neuroinflammation. Inflammatory processes in the brain and spinal cord may contribute to the cognitive difficulties—sometimes referred to as "brain fog"—that affect many patients. Discerning the nature and extent of neuroinflammation is an active area of investigation that could lead to targeted anti-inflammatory strategies.

Lastly, new imaging techniques and biomarker discovery are accelerating the pace of research. Sophisticated scans can now visualize areas of the brain that process pain and fatigue, offering insights into their functioning in the context of CFS and FM. Meanwhile, identifying reliable biomarkers can help in the diagnostic process, offering quantifiable indicators of the conditions to supplement the somewhat subjective symptom reports.

In summary, the scientific study of CFS and FM is entering an exciting era. With an arsenal of innovative research techniques and a growing acknowledgment of the complexity of these disorders, we're on the cusp of substantial breakthroughs. These insights won't just deepen our understanding—they'll empower patients and practitioners alike with more effective tools for managing and overcoming the challenges of these conditions.

By recognizing your body's unique patterns and contributing factors, keeping abreast of research developments, and maintaining open lines of communication with healthcare providers, you can navigate the complexities of CFS and FM with greater resolve. Each new discovery brings us closer to delivering tangible relief and reclaiming the quality of life that every individual deserves.

Chapter 3:
Personal Stories of Resilience

In the heart of the struggle with Chronic Fatigue Syndrome (CFS) and Fibromyalgia (FM), it can be tremendously empowering to know that you're not alone. Chapter 3 uncovers the deeply personal journeys of those who've navigated the turbulent waters of these chronic illnesses. Through a rich tapestry of firsthand accounts, you'll find not just stories of the hardships and setbacks that come with CFS and FM, but vivid narratives that speak to the human spirit's incredible capacity for resilience. Salted with laughter and tears, these sagas of survival connect you to a community that stands defiantly in the face of their condition. You'll witness the transformation from despair to hope as individuals share hard-won victories and the lessons learned along the road to recovery. It's within these stories that the true depth of human perseverance shines—as one's darkest moments often give birth to a newfound strength—providing solace and a silent whisper to carry on when you need it most.

Living with Chronic Illness: Firsthand Accounts

The road that stretches before those living with chronic conditions like Chronic Fatigue Syndrome (CFS) and Fibromyalgia (FM) is often winding and treacherous. It's easy to feel isolated in such a journey, but woven through the silence are threads of shared humanity, strands of stories that connect individuals facing similar tribulations. These narratives aren't just tales of struggles; they are powerful testaments of the resilience that emanates from the human spirit.

There's something uniquely profound about hearing from someone who's walked the path you're treading. The narratives from those with CFS and FM offer insights that are at once familiar and eye-opening. They speak of the initial confusion upon encountering unrelenting exhaustion, the frustration of aches that eluded explanation, and the cascade of emotions these symptoms unleashed.

Listening to these firsthand accounts, you begin to piece together the broader tapestry of life with chronic illness. There's the story of a once-active individual, whose life was turned upside-down by an invisible force; they had to learn to celebrate the small victories, such as taking a shower or making dinner, which pre-illness wouldn't have even registered as achievements.

Or consider the parent who had to navigate the intricacies of care both for their children and themselves, juggling the guilt of being unable to participate fully in their kids' lives with the necessity of self-care. Through trial and error, they discovered the delicate balance between pushing their limits and listening to their body's pleas for rest.

Then there's the narrative of the young professional whose burgeoning career felt threatened by an onslaught of inexplicable symptoms. Despite the uncertainty, they crafted a routine that embraced flexible work hours and remote engagements, allowing them to remain an active part of the workforce.

Each story is a tile in the larger mosaic of chronic illness. Patterns emerge: the importance of self-advocacy, the significant role of compassionate healthcare providers, and the invaluable support of friends and family. But no less vital are the personal strategies that individuals developed to manage their symptoms. From meticulous pacing to adapting hobbies, these stories are rich with coping mechanisms.

In these accounts, the concept of pain takes on new dimensions. Beyond the physical discomfort, there's the emotional toll of being misunderstood by those who can't see the pain. The need for validation is a recurrent theme, and it's through connection with others that many find solace and strength to persist.

Fatigue, too, is explored in depth—the all-consuming kind that isn't alleviated by sleep. Here, the conventional wisdom of "more rest equals more energy" often doesn't apply. Instead, people living with CFS and FM recount learning how to apportion their energy judiciously, like a precious resource, honoring their body's rhythms and needs.

The battle against the dual specters of skepticism and disbelief is also chronicled. In these stories, the invisible nature of CFS and FM is a significant adversary. Much of the fight involves proving the reality of their experiences, not only to doubting acquaintances but sometimes to healthcare professionals as well.

Amid the recollections of hardship, however, there is hope. Moments of profound connection, as one finds a supportive community, turn the tide of isolation. There's talk of finding joy in the simplicity of a moment's relief, or the unexpected kindness of a stranger who offers understanding instead of judgment.

Stories of resilience are peppered with pragmatic tips, like keeping a symptoms journal, which has helped many to communicate effectively with their doctors. Or employing creative visualization techniques, which provide a mental escape hatch on days when physical pain confines them.

There's wisdom in these lived experiences, knowledge that is often hard-earned and deeply personal. For every individual who shares their story, there's an unspoken acknowledgment that their journey might light the way for another.

Ultimately, these firsthand accounts weave a narrative of enduring, not merely surviving, with chronic illness. They display a peculiar kind of bravery that comes from facing each day's uncertainty with a heart full of hope. They inspire others to find their coping strategies, and perhaps most importantly, to keep sustaining the belief that life, although different, can still be meaningful and full of possibilities.

As the stories unfold, an unseen community forms, a gathering of kindred spirits who, despite never having met, are intimately connected through shared experiences. They're a reminder that while everyone's journey is unique, no one has to walk the path alone, and together, the path becomes a little less daunting, a little more infused with hope.

The collective wisdom of those who speak of lives intertwined with chronic illness does not claim to offer a cure or a one-size-fits-all solution. What it does provide is a testament to the human spirit's ability to adapt, to find happiness in the face of chronic illness, and to cultivate an environment where wellbeing, however redefined, can flourish.

From Despair to Hope: Recovery Narratives

Each journey through the terrain of chronic illness is uniquely challenging, marked with moments of despair and stretches of stony silence where hope seems a distant echo. Yet, with resilience and courage, those with Chronic Fatigue Syndrome and Fibromyalgia carve paths to recovery that are as inspiring as they are instructive. These narratives are not merely stories; they are lifelines of insight for anyone seeking solace and solutions amidst the struggles of chronic illness.

Imagine the unrelenting grip of fatigue that sinks its teeth deep into your daily life, where even the simplest tasks transform into mountains. This is the relentless reality for many grappling with CFS and FM. It's a reality that John, a 45-year old teacher, knows all too well. His narrative begins with feeling disconsolate upon diagnosis, worried about his future, how he would manage his career, his passion for travel, and even his ability to engage in simple joys like playing with his kids.

For Laura, a 30-year old graphics designer, the despair sank in as she grappled with the invisible chains of these conditions, feeling misunderstood by friends and colleagues who couldn't see her pain. She describes the journey out of despair as one paved with patience, self-compassion, and the gradual collection of small victories. The transformation isn't abrupt; it's kindled over time, with each day a bit brighter than the last.

Edward's tale is one of transformation too, where latent creativity became central to his healing process. Before CFS and FM, he never imagined that painting would become his sanctuary, a place where his body's limitations didn't define his existence. He talks about the therapeutic effects of color and form, something that carried him through the toughest times.

Then there's Sofia, whose narrative is tinged with the complexities of motherhood intersecting chronic illness. Each step towards recovery was balanced with the nurturing of her children, and her story illustrates how the love for her family fueled her determination to find wellness amidst the turmoil. Her journey showcases the power of an indomitable spirit and the strength that comes from caring for others.

Recalling soul-wrenching moments of solitude, Mia shares how she turned to nature for solace. The validation she sought wasn't found in the countless doctor's offices but rather in the quiet whispers of the wind and the ceaseless waves of the ocean that promised continuity and a sense of peace.

Part of moving from despair to hope is learning and leveraging. For Caleb, it was the meticulous chronicling of his experiences—detailing what exacerbated his symptoms and what relieved them—that pioneered his road to recovery. He became an investigator in his own life story, leaving no stone unturned in his quest to reclaim his vitality.

Amid these testimonials, one universal truth emerges: recovery narratives are not linear. They meander like rivers, sometimes lost beneath the surface, other times breaking through with clarity and momentum. Alexis's story emphasizes this ebb and flow, as she recounts the days of profound exhaustion and unexpected resurgence—both holding space in her recovery.

An element often woven into the tapestry of these narratives is the importance of community and connection. For Darnell, it was a support group composed of fellow warriors battling CFS and FM that became his lifeline. Within this community, despair was met with understanding and practical advice, transforming isolation into shared determination.

While many of these stories reflect personal resilience, they also underscore the significant role of healthcare providers. Lily speaks of a particularly empathetic doctor who became a beacon of hope, guiding her through the haze of uncertainty with an informed, yet heartfelt approach to treatment.

There are also testimonies that reveal how advocacy plays an integral part in the journey from desolation to hopefulness. When Mark felt dismissed by the medical community, he took it upon himself to become an articulate spokesperson for his own health, demanding and acquiring the attention and respect he needed to move forward.

The rippling impact of attitude adjustment is another vibrant thread in these stories. Sarah's epiphany that her mindset could either be her prison or her wings brought about a pivotal shift in her recovery. Celebrating mini-triumphs and reframing setbacks as opportunities for growth became her mantra.

Bridging these diverse experiences is the embrace of holistic approaches to health. For instance, Zach found balance through an integrated regime involving both conventional and alternative therapies, recognizing that healing often requires a symphony of interventions—each instrument playing a critical part in the harmony of health.

The journey of recovery isn't reserved for the sufferer alone. We find in these chronicles that caregivers, too, experience their own evolution. Sophia recounts the ways in which caring for her husband transformed her own perceptions of health, compassion, and the importance of togetherness in the face of chronic illness.

Conclusively, these narratives illuminate the resilience of the human spirit. They exemplify the transition from a disillusioned acceptance of chronic illness to an emboldened reclamation of life. It's a journey marked by gradual successes sewn together by persistence and fortitude, a journey from despair to hope that offers a profound message: within the folds of our challenges lies the potential for profound transformation and healing.

As these narratives unfurl, they weave a fabric of inspiration for anyone navigating the tempest of CFS and FM. They remind us all that while the path may be fraught with obstacles, it is also dotted with possibility, and through shared experiences, we find not only solace but also strategies for a hopeful and healthier tomorrow.

Chapter 4:
Nutrition and Diet: Fueling Your Path to Wellness

Embarking upon the road to wellness, nutrition takes a front seat as an empowering ally for those grappling with Chronic Fatigue Syndrome and Fibromyalgia. Let's delve into the symbiotic relationship between what we eat and how we feel, unraveling the intricate tapestry of nutrients that could help recharge your body's depleted energy stores. This chapter isn't just about listing foods; it's about understanding the profound impact that a thoughtful, well-curated diet can have on dampening inflammation and nourishing your body's every cell. We'll explore how embracing an anti-inflammatory lifestyle may not just quell the embers of chronic illness but can be the spark that reignites the vibrancy of life. Navigating through the maze of dietary advice can be overwhelming, but we're here to arm you with knowledge and strategies so that you can tailor a diet that resonates with your body's unique needs. Think of this as your culinary compass, guiding you to make choices that fuel your journey to wellness with the most potent of medicines: the food on your plate.

Essential Nutrients and Supplements for CFS and FM

Navigating the maze of nutrition when dealing with Chronic Fatigue Syndrome (CFS) and Fibromyalgia (FM) can be daunting, but understanding the role of essential nutrients and supplements is a beacon of light on this journey. Though no one-size-fits-all regimen exists, there are certain nutritional keystones known to fortify the body. Magnesium, for instance, often runs on empty in those with FM and CFS, and bolstering levels can help ease muscle pain and improve sleep. Together with the right balance of Omega-3 fatty acids, known for their anti-inflammatory properties, and Coenzyme Q10 to boost energy production at a cellular level, you're equipping your body's arsenal to fend off the daily battles of fatigue and discomfort. Choosing high-quality, bioavailable forms of vitamins B12 and D, as each play critical roles – the former in neurological function and energy, the latter in immune health and possibly pain reduction. Dreaming of a day without the heavy cloak of tiredness or the sharp bite of aching muscles starts with these small, yet potent, allies. As you weave these essentials into the fabric of your daily nutrition, remember to be patient with your body and celebrate the small victories – for each step forward is a step toward wellness.

Vitamins and Minerals play a nuanced role in tackling the complexities of Chronic Fatigue Syndrome (CFS) and Fibromyalgia (FM). Just as the gears of a watch work synchronously to tell time, vitamins and minerals work together within your body to maintain health and support recovery. For individuals experiencing CFS and FM, the balance of these vital nutrients can sometimes tip – with even a minor deficiency potentially exacerbating symptoms or hindering recovery.

Sufficient intake of **Vitamin D**, often hailed as the 'sunshine vitamin', is crucial. A deficiency in Vitamin D is not uncommon in cases of CFS and FM. It's imperative to have your levels tested and if they're low, supplementation may be a necessary step in your wellness journey. Adequate Vitamin D aids in immune function and muscle repair – both areas of concern when dealing with these conditions.

Similarly, the B-Vitamin family – particularly **Vitamin B12** and **Folate (B9)** – has been linked with improved energy levels and cognitive function. Oral supplementation or even injections of Vitamin B12, under professional guidance, have been reported to ease fatigue for many.

Another key player is **Magnesium**. This mineral is like the body's natural chill pill, involved in over 300 biochemical reactions. From muscle relaxation to improved sleep, optimizing magnesium levels through dietary sources or supplements might be a game-changer for those with muscle pains and insomnia associated with CFS and FM.

Let's not forget about **Iron**. Given that iron is essential for transporting oxygen in the blood, any deficit can leave you feeling tired and short of breath. It's important, though, to confirm with a physician before starting iron supplements, as too much can be harmful.

Investigating your **Zinc** status may also be worthwhile. Zinc plays a multifaceted role in immune function, enzyme reactions, and DNA synthesis – areas that can be under pressure in CFS and FM. Zinc's ability to support immune health is vital, considering how these conditions can potentially root from or cause immune system disruptions.

The sea mineral **Iodine** is central to thyroid function, which governs metabolism. An underactive thyroid - also common in CFS and FM - can mirror many symptoms of these conditions, such as fatigue and joint/muscle pain. Monitoring and maintaining proper iodine intake can sometimes improve symptom management.

Antioxidant vitamins like **Vitamin C** and **Vitamin E** take on added significance given their role in protecting the body against oxidative stress and aiding in tissue repair – particularly helpful when your body is under the constant strain of chronic illness.

Let's circle back to energy. The mineral **Coenzyme Q10 (CoQ10)**, which is actually considered a vitamin-like substance, supports energy production at the cellular level. With energy in such short supply for CFS and FM sufferers, ensuring you're not running low on CoQ10 could be part of a wider strategy to replenish your energy reserves.

The importance of **Calcium** goes beyond bone health. It helps regulate nerve transmission and muscle function, which can be beneficial when muscle spasms or neuropathic pain are part of your symptom complex. Pairing calcium with Vitamin D and magnesium ensures better absorption and utilization.

When we talk about the nervous system, **Potassium** steps up as it is imperative for nerve function and muscle control. A proper balance between Potassium and Sodium is crucial for those fighting CFS and FM, especially due to the potential for dysregulation of cellular transport and nerve signaling.

We must also spotlight **Selenium**, an often-overlooked mineral that acts as a powerful antioxidant and supports thyroid function. Balancing selenium intake can be a delicate process but worth investigating, particularly if you're experiencing ongoing fatigue and muscle weakness.

Your antioxidant defense system leans heavily on the mineral **Manganese**, which can help fend off the free radical damage commonly associated with chronic conditions like CFS and FM. Manganese also supports the metabolism of cholesterol, carbohydrates, and protein – processes that often need extra support in these conditions.

To wrap up our microscopic tour, the trace mineral **Molybdenum** is also essential for various biochemical reactions in the body, even though required in minute quantities. Being vigilant about such details can sometimes untangle the knotted symptoms of CFS and FM.

All this talk about vitamins and minerals might make you wonder about the best path to balance them – diets, supplements, or a mix of both? Well, it is individual. Some may absorb nutrients well from their diet/supplements, others may not due to gut issues common in CFS/FM. It's essential to work with a healthcare provider to tailor a regime that fits your body's unique needs.

Integrating a well-rounded approach that respects the distinctiveness of your body's needs is key. Through careful monitoring, you can utilize vitamins and nutrients not only to nourish but to help rebuild and sustain the processes that keep you moving forward on your path to wellness.

Probiotics and Digestive Enzymes

As we continue to explore effective nutritional strategies for managing Chronic Fatigue Syndrome (CFS) and Fibromyalgia (FM), it's essential to understand the role of gut health and digestion in overall wellness. The gut is often referred to as the "second brain," and for a good reason. It's home to a complex and delicate ecosystem of bacteria and enzymes that play a crucial role in processing the food you eat, absorbing nutrients, and managing immune responses. Now, let's delve into how probiotics and digestive enzymes may fit into the puzzle of managing symptoms associated with CFS and FM.

The term "probiotics" refers to beneficial bacteria that inhabit our digestive tract. These microscopic allies are vital in maintaining the intestinal barrier, outcompeting harmful pathogens, and supporting optimal immune function. For individuals battling CFS and FM, probiotics can be particularly helpful in managing gastrointestinal symptoms which are all too common with these conditions.

So, how do probiotics work to your advantage? Picture your gut flora as a lush garden - when it's well-cared-for, it's less likely to be overrun by weeds, or in this case, harmful bacteria. Adding probiotics can replenish and sustain the right balance of beneficial bacteria in your gut. They assist in digestion, reduce inflammation, and may even help alleviate some of the exhausting symptoms you're facing.

However, navigating the world of probiotics can be a touch overwhelming. With so many strains and varieties available, selecting the right one could seem like a daunting task. The key, though, is to look for a high-quality product with a variety of well-researched strains, and, when in doubt, consulting with a healthcare professional savvy in CFS/FM can provide guidance tailored to your specific needs.

Now, let's shift gears to digestive enzymes. They are powerful proteins that break down food into absorbable components, making it possible for your body to access the nutrients locked within the food you consume. When your body doesn't secrete enough of these enzymes naturally, as is often the case with CFS/FM, you might experience bloating, gas, or discomfort after meals. Thus, supplemental digestive enzymes can step in as valuable assistants in the digestion process.

Including enzymes in your regimen can result in better nutrient absorption and less gastrointestinal distress, which in turn can aid in reducing overall fatigue and discomfort. It's much like giving your digestive system a helping hand, easing its workload so your body can focus on using energy in other vital areas – perhaps healing and managing symptoms.

A combination of proteases (which break down proteins), lipases (for fats), and amylases (for carbohydrates) is typically what you'll find in a full-spectrum enzyme supplement. These could potentially bring significant relief, especially during flare-ups or times when your digestive system seems particularly sluggish.

Remember, everyone's microbiome is unique, so what works wonders for one person may not work the same way for you. This is a journey of trial, patience, and attentiveness to your body's responses. Start low with dose and go slow – introducing new supplements gradually to monitor your body's reactions.

Amidst managing CFS and FM, it can be easy to underestimate the importance of gut health. But let me assure you, this avenue of health is not one to overlook. An unhappy gut can be a significant source of irritation, exacerbating both the weariness and discomfort associated with these conditions. Addressing digestive health with probiotics and enzymes can sometimes provide relief in ways you might not have considered possible.

Here's something to chew on – not only can probiotics and enzymes assist with digestion, but they also play a role in synthesizing certain vitamins and battling inflammation. This is particularly relevant because vitamin deficiencies and systemic inflammation could be ongoing battles with CFS and FM.

It's essential to remember that these supplements are not a magic bullet. They're a single part of a multifaceted approach to managing CFS and FM. Diet, sleep, exercise, stress management, and medications or other supplements will all likely feature in your personalized plan for wellness.

Incorporating probiotics and digestive enzymes might require some adjustments along the way. Noticing subtle differences in how you feel on a day-to-day basis is key. It's about being in tune with your body and the small signals it gives as it responds to the changes you make. This heightened self-awareness will serve you well on your journey to wellness.

Moving forward with probiotics and enzymes is indicative of a broader principle in managing CFS and FM: the value of nurturing our internal ecosystem. As we support the intricate network inside, it's just as important to cultivate our external ecosystems - our environments, relationships, and lifestyle choices. Everything is interconnected in the grander scope of health and healing.

In conclusion, while the world of probiotics and digestive enzymes may seem complex, the potential benefits these supplements offer for individuals dealing with CFS and FM make them worth consideration. By supporting digestive health, you may find improvements in areas such as energy levels, immune function, and overall well-being. Be patient with the process, open to adjustment, and, most importantly, compassionate with yourself as you navigate this path. Your journey to wellness is just that - uniquely yours. With each small step, you are potentially moving closer to a life of more comfort, vitality, and joy.

Recommended Foods and Anti-Inflammatory Diet Tips

When embarking on a wellness journey, particularly with conditions like Chronic Fatigue Syndrome (CFS) and Fibromyalgia (FM), one of the most transformative areas we can explore is our diet. The power of an anti-inflammatory diet is undeniable, and tuning into foods that nourish rather than inflame can be a game-changer.

First and foremost, incorporating a rainbow of vegetables into your meals is a way to guarantee you're getting a plethora of nutrients and antioxidants that combat inflammation. Leafy greens, such as spinach and kale, are nutritional powerhouses, rich in vitamins and minerals that support overall health.

Fatty fish, like salmon, sardines, and mackerel, are excellent sources of Omega-3 fatty acids, which have strong anti-inflammatory properties. Twice-weekly servings of these can help manage inflammation and pain associated with CFS and FM.

Fruits can also play an important role; berries, cherries, and apples are particularly beneficial due to their high antioxidant content. However, it's important to balance fruit intake with your body's needs, as excessive sugar, even from natural sources, can lead to energy crashes.

Including whole grains in your diet is another way to ensure you're fueling your body adequately. Options like quinoa, brown rice, and oats are not only filling but also high in fiber, which can improve digestive health—a common concern among those with CFS and FM.

Nuts and seeds, such as almonds, walnuts, chia seeds, and flaxseeds, are not only great snacks but also important sources of good fats and can help reduce inflammation.

Beans and legumes are also key players. They provide protein, fiber, and a range of nutrients, and are incredibly versatile in meals, from soups to salads to main dishes.

Healthy fats are essential; utilizing olive oil for cooking or in dressings can provide the benefits of mono-unsaturated fats. Embracing avocados, whether in guacamole or as a toast topper, can also boost your intake of these good fats.

Spices are nature's pharmacy and can deeply enhance the anti-inflammatory power of your meals. Turmeric, ginger, cinnamon, and garlic not only add flavor but also have medicinal qualities that can help reduce inflammation and boost immunity.

It's also beneficial to hydrate adequately with water throughout the day. Proper hydration aids digestion, nutrient absorption, and energy levels—all crucial for managing CFS and FM.

Probiotic-rich foods such as yogurt, kefir, and sauerkraut can support gut health. A healthy gut flora has been linked to reduced systemic inflammation and better immune function, which may alleviate some symptoms of CFS and FM.

When it comes to beverages, green tea is particularly beneficial. It contains epigallocatechin gallate (EGCG), an antioxidant that has been shown to reduce inflammation and support health.

For those with a sweet tooth, opting for dark chocolate with a high cocoa content can be gratifying. In moderation, this treat provides antioxidants that can help fight inflammation, just be mindful of the sugar content.

What's as important as the foods you include is what you might consider reducing or avoiding. Processed foods, excessive sugars, and unhealthy fats can all contribute to inflammation and exacerbate symptoms of CFS and FM. Identifying any personal food sensitivities is also key, as they can silently contribute to inflammation.

Last but not least, remember to listen to your body—it's your ultimate guide. Incorporating an anti-inflammatory diet doesn't mean a one-size-fits-all approach. It's about finding balance, enjoying food, and observing how your body responds. Small, gradual changes are more sustainable than drastic overhauls. And with every meal, you're investing in a foundation of wellness that can support you on this journey.

Chapter 5:
Managing Pain and Fatigue

As we delve into the heart of our journey—the crux of what so many are yearning to conquer—we turn a keen eye to managing the twin towers of challenge in chronic conditions: pain and fatigue. Here, nestled within these pages, lies a mosaic of strategies designed to arm you with the knowledge to reclaim your life's narrative. Grappling with the relentless grip of discomfort and exhaustion can feel like an uphill battle, but empowerment begins with understanding that there's a spectrum of tools at your disposal. We unfurl a tapestry of techniques that range from honing in on your body's natural pain relief mechanisms to harnessing the elegance of pacing—an art form that balances activity with restorative breaks. Break the cycle of push and crash by tuning into your own rhythmic ebb and flow, and learn to navigate your days with grace and endurance. This chapter is not about quick fixes but about cultivating a sustainable harmony within your life's symphony. Consider each option as a potential ally in your quest, recognizing that it's okay to navigate this part of your journey at your own pace, one mindful step at a time.

Pain Management Strategies

Embarking on the journey towards managing chronic pain is both a challenge and an empowerment. It's about matchmaking your body's needs with the symphony of strategies at your disposal. When your muscles feel like they're wrapped in barbed wire, pharmaceutical interventions can sometimes be a tender mercy, easing the raw edges of your discomfort. But let's not overlook the powerhouse of non-pharmaceutical therapies that cast a wide net of relief: think gentle yoga that unfolds your pain, mindful meditation that calms the stormy seas of aching limbs, or acupuncture's precise pinpricks re-routing your pain pathways. It's about finding that sacred balance where managing pain becomes less about fierce battles and more about harmonious truces. As you flip through the following pages, remember, pain management is personal, dynamic, and adjustive. It isn't just a list of remedies; it's an art form where you paint over the canvas of pain with strokes of resilience, patience, and self-compassion.

Pharmaceutical Options

As we explore the landscape of pain and fatigue management techniques, it becomes evident that in some cases, medication may complement your wellness plan. Living with Chronic Fatigue Syndrome (CFS) and Fibromyalgia (FM) can be akin to navigating an ever-shifting labyrinth, and pharmaceuticals often serve as a vital tool in your arsenal.

For those coping with the daily reality of CFS and FM, pain might range from a dull ache to a searing, ever-present sensation. Understandably, pain relief becomes a top priority. Analgesics, including over-the-counter options like acetaminophen and NSAIDs (non-steroidal anti-inflammatory drugs), might be recommended for handling mild pain. However, these should be used judiciously, considering potential side effects and the risk of over-reliance.

Opioids are another category of pain medication. They can be indispensable for short-term relief but are prescribed with caution due to risks like dependency and tolerance. It's crucial to have a frank dialogue with your healthcare provider about the benefits and risks, ensuring that if opioids are part of your treatment, you're both diligent about monitoring their use.

Perhaps less known are medications such as antidepressants – not just for their mood-stabilizing properties but also because certain types can ease pain and improve sleep. Tricyclic antidepressants, for example, have a track record of helping some patients with FM to attain a deeper level of restorative sleep which can, in turn, reduce pain.

Anticonvulsants, traditionally used to treat epilepsy, may also have a place in your management regimen. Their ability to calm nerve impulses might lead to diminished pain. Drugs like pregabalin (Lyrica) and gabapentin (Neurontin) are commonly used with various degrees of success and are important to consider if your pain has a pronounced nerve-based component.

For the all-encompassing fatigue that is synonymous with CFS and FM, stimulant medications like modafinil (Provigil) might be indicated. Though they can't tackle the underlying cause of tiredness, they may help manage its symptoms, allowing for periods of increased alertness and activity. However, remember that these are not long-term solutions and should be used strategically.

Muscle relaxants can sometimes offer temporary relief from muscle pain and spasms, a typical grievance for FM sufferers. However, their sedative effect can complicate fatigue issues, meaning their use needs to be carefully balanced for effectiveness without exacerbating tiredness.

Another significant aspect of medication management involves addressing secondary symptoms such as irritable bowel syndrome or migraines, which often accompany CFS and FM. Targeted medications can provide relief and improve overall quality of life, making day-to-day experiences more bearable.

Some patients find that hormone replacement therapy, particularly addressing thyroid issues, adrenal insufficiency, or sex hormone imbalances, can alleviate some of the symptoms associated with CFS and FM. These therapies should be pursued under close supervision, ensuring that your unique physiological needs are met.

A note on medication tolerance – your body's response can change over time. What works for you initially may require adjustments down the road. This is where the partnership with your healthcare provider is essential, ensuring that your treatment evolves with your condition.

It's also paramount to consider drug interactions, especially if you are dealing with multiple prescriptions. Each new medication brings a risk of interaction with your current regimen that could negate benefits or, worse, cause harm. Always check with a pharmacist or doctor before adding anything new to your medication routine.

And let's not overlook the importance of tracking your symptoms and medication effects. Keeping a detailed log can help you and your care team pinpoint what medications offer relief and which may incur unwanted side effects. Knowledge is power, and this knowledge empowers you to take charge of your treatment.

While much of this journey involves trial and error, the goal is to find a pharmaceutical balance that boosts your overall well-being. This means managing side effects and avoiding medication overtreatment, which can sometimes occur in a well-intentioned bid to chase away the pain and fatigue.

Ultimately, the pursuit of the right medication is an exercise in hope and persistence. Many people with CFS and FM have walked this path and found a measure of relief. Be patient with yourself and remain in constant communication with those dedicated to helping you navigate these options.

Remember, though, while pharmaceuticals can offer respite, they are best used as part of a comprehensive approach, which might include dietary modifications, lifestyle changes, and complementary therapies. In the harmonious fusion of these strategies often lies the tranquility that so many with CFS and FM seek.

In summary, the world of pharmaceuticals is broad and diverse, offering many avenues of potential relief. But it is not without its complexities and pitfalls. It's essential to proceed with careful consideration, informed decisions, and unflagging optimism as you find the path that's best for you.

Non-Pharmaceutical Therapies

Now take center stage as we explore a variety of methods to manage the symptoms of Chronic Fatigue Syndrome (CFS) and Fibromyalgia (FM). For many, the path to wellness includes treatments beyond medication, employing holistic strategies that touch every aspect of one's life.

First and foremost, managing these conditions often calls for a multidisciplinary approach. Engaging in cognitive behavioral therapy and mindfulness, which we'll delve deeper into in later sections, are cornerstones of non-pharmaceutical interventions. However, there's a whole tool kit at your disposal that can complement these methods and potentially enhance your quality of life.

One major area of interest for many is the use of graded exercise therapy (GET). The key is to start low and go slow, gradually increasing physical activity within one's own tolerance. Patients have found that activities such as walking, swimming, or tai chi can not only improve stamina but also reduce pain over time. It's crucial, however, to monitor your symptoms and ensure you're not exacerbating them.

Pain can be unrelenting, but that doesn't mean relief is out of reach. Physical therapy, employing techniques like myofascial release and gentle stretching, can alleviate some of the discomfort. Therapists adept in these areas can also provide individualized plans to strengthen the body without overexerting it.

Biofeedback and neurofeedback are also promising areas. These techniques harness the power of your mind to influence bodily functions, like heart rate and muscle tension, which may be out of whack in CFS and FM. It's a method that fosters self-regulation and bolsters responses to stress and pain.

Speaking of the mind, let's not forget the immense benefits of relaxation techniques. Deep breathing exercises, progressive muscle relaxation, or visualization can transport you to a state of calm, providing ample respite from the daily stressors that may exacerbate your symptoms.

The ancient practice of acupuncture also offers a needle of hope. Many find that this time-honored therapy, which focuses on various pressure points in the body, can improve pain and overall well-being. While it might not work for everyone, its benefit for some can be striking and worth a trial if you're looking for alternatives.

Massage therapy goes hand in hand with acupuncture. Its soothing strokes offer not just physical relief but also emotional solace by reducing stress. Importantly, finding a therapist experienced with CFS and FM is key; they'll understand the nuances of your condition and tailor their technique accordingly.

A less conventional option includes the use of transcutaneous electrical nerve stimulation (TENS). These devices send small electrical currents to the body's nerve endings, potentially easing pain. It's non-invasive, and while some may shrug it off, others swear by its efficacy.

Yoga and Pilates are not just trends; they bring a bounty of benefits for those with chronic conditions. Their emphasis on breathing, alignment, and controlled movements makes them an ideal choice for managing symptoms. Many have discovered that these practices enhance flexibility, control, and even emotional well-being.

Proper nutrition plays a vital role and deserves its own spotlight. An anti-inflammatory diet may ease symptoms, and while we touch upon diet in a different chapter, it's important to reiterate its role in the non-pharmaceutical realm. What you put into your body impacts how you feel, so it's worthwhile to consider dietary changes as part of your therapy.

Hydrotherapy and balneotherapy, which involve the use of water for pain relief and improving physical function, can also be soothing. Whether it's a warm bath at home or a directed therapy at a specialized facility, the power of water shouldn't be underestimated.

Less recognized but increasingly popular are artistic therapies. Engaging in music, art, or writing can offer a cathartic outlet for your emotions, reduce stress, and serve as a means for expression when words fall short. The meditative state these activities inspire may also relieve symptoms for some.

Chiropractic care, though often associated with spinal adjustments, can extend beyond that. With a practitioner skilled in addressing CFS and FM issues, this therapy can improve range of motion and reduce pain, sometimes significantly contributing to a patient's comfort.

Lastly, it's important to acknowledge the role emotional and spiritual well-being play in managing CFS and FM. Incorporating practices that address these aspects – perhaps through community involvement, faith, or meditation – can make an instrumental difference in coping with these conditions. This whole-body approach to health isn't just about treating symptoms but nurturing oneself wholly.

While none of these therapies may be a cure, they offer a spectrum of hope – options and opportunities to reclaim bits of your life and find relief on your terms. Empower yourself by exploring these non-pharmaceutical avenues; you may discover that the keys to managing your symptoms lie in the harmony of body, mind, and spirit.

Energy Conservation and Pacing Techniques

As we venture further into the realm of managing chronic fatigue syndrome (CFS) and fibromyalgia (FM), it's vital to recognize that tending to energy is as crucial as managing pain. The concept of energy conservation and pacing isn't about restricting life but rather embracing it with a new, thoughtful approach. It's about finding balance; the sweet spot between activity and rest that allows you to sustain a stable level of functioning over time. Think of it as a budgeting exercise where energy is your currency—you need to spend it wisely to avoid bankruptcy.

Firstly, let's demystify pacing: it's the art of spacing out activities to avoid peaks and valleys in your energy levels. Pacing is not a one-size-fits-all solution; it's a personalized strategy. Understanding your body's signals and respecting your energy limits is fundamental. Start by gauging your daily energy levels—keep a diary if you must. Note the times when you're feeling more alert and those when you're not. Scheduling demanding tasks during your natural high-energy windows can maximize your effectiveness.

Learning to say no can be liberating. Chronic illness often instills a sense of guilt for being unable to keep up with demands, but it's crucial to set boundaries. Accepting your limits is not admitting defeat—it's an act of self-care. So, when you're running low on energy, it's perfectly okay to decline additional responsibilities. Remember, by conserving your energy, you're ensuring you're there for the most crucial moments.

Breaking up tasks into smaller, manageable chunks is another effective technique. Instead of attempting to tackle a huge project in one go, split it up and intersperse it with short rest periods. This method, also known as time-based pacing, helps to prevent overexertion. Consider rest as a strategic move, not a retreat. These mini-breaks are your checkpoints, allowing you to recharge and reset.

An often overlooked, yet significant aspect of energy conservation, lies in the environment within which you operate. Organize your living and working spaces for efficiency. Keep commonly used items within easy reach, and ensure that your environment supports your ability to function with minimal strain. Simple changes, like comfortable seating or a well-arranged room, can conserve energy that would otherwise be spent on unnecessary physical exertion.

The concept of 'energy envelopes' is a practical visual tool you can use. Picture your energy as an envelope of resources you get each day. It can't be overstuffed without consequences, nor can you borrow from tomorrow's envelope. Distributing your energy envelope evenly throughout the day, dedicating portions to different activities, allows for a balanced approach to daily living.

Mindfulness practices can enhance energy conservation by bringing your attention to the present moment, helping you recognize early fatigue signs. By tuning into your body's cues, you can better pace your activities and rest before hitting the point of exhaustion. Mindful breathing or meditation can serve as calming techniques during rest periods, enriching the quality of your breaks.

Delegating tasks is another form of energy conservation. It involves letting go of the idea that you must do everything yourself. Enlist help for more physically demanding chores, or consider automating or using assistive devices to ease the burden.

Next, prioritize your activities. Distinguish between what's necessary, what's important, and what's optional. The necessary tasks demand your energy first, while the optional ones can wait. By prioritizing, you ensure that your limited energy is spent on what truly matters to you.

When dealing with CFS and FM, anticipate fluctuations in your energy levels. Having a flexible plan that can adapt to your changing energy landscapes is critical. On days when your energy is higher than usual, resist the urge to go full throttle; conversely, on low-energy days, permit yourself to take it easy without self-judgment.

Energy conservation is not only about managing physical tasks; it's also about managing emotional and social energies. Emotional stress can be incredibly draining and learning stress management techniques is an essential part of conserving your energy. Similarly, engaging in social activities necessitates energy expenditure. Be selective about the events you attend and don't hesitate to excuse yourself for a breather when needed.

It's important to embrace assistive technologies and adaptive devices designed to make life easier. These tools can significantly reduce physical strain and conserve energy. From ergonomic furniture to voice recognition software, there's a plethora of tools available that can ease the burden of daily tasks.

Resting before you're exhausted may sound counterintuitive, but it's an effective pacing technique. It's easier to recuperate from a level of mild fatigue than from complete exhaustion. Proactive rest can help maintain a more consistent energy level throughout the day.

Finally, cultivate patience. The culture of instant gratification and constant hustle can make pacing seem unproductive, but it's important to remind yourself that pacing is a long game. It requires patience, persistent practice, and persistence, qualities that will serve you well on your wellness journey.

In essence, energy conservation and pacing are about respecting your body's needs, consciously choosing how to expend your energy, and making modifications to maintain a life that is as full and satisfying as possible. By implementing these strategies, you'll be better positioned to manage pain and fatigue, paving the way to a more enjoyable and sustainable day-to-day existence.

Chapter 6:
The Role of Sleep in Healing

Sleep isn't just a break from the daily grind; it's a critical ally in the healing journey for those grappling with Chronic Fatigue Syndrome and Fibromyalgia. As we fold the page on strategies for managing pain and fatigue, let's dim the lights on another restorative facet: sleep. This silent healer works behind the scenes, orchestrating a symphony of physiological repairs that the weary bodies of CFS and FM patients yearn for. Now, imagine your bedroom transforming into a sanctuary where sleep, no longer elusive, cocoons you into its restorative embrace. Look beyond counting sheep; we're talking about nurturing sleep environments, embracing routines that signal your brain it's time to unwind, and fostering patterns that invite uninterrupted cycles of deep, healing sleep. It's about time we tuned into our body's natural rhythms, giving ourselves permission to prioritize rest and acknowledge the restorative power of a good night's sleep in our recovery repertoire. It's about embracing the darkness to bring forth the light of better days, fueled by the rejuvenating force of slumber. This chapter opens the doorway to nights of rejuvenated dreams, setting the stage for restoration at cellular levels, and ultimately, threading the golden strand of sleep into the fabric of your wellness tapestry.

Understanding Sleep Dysfunctions in CFS and FM

As we delve into the intricacies of healing from Chronic Fatigue Syndrome (CFS) and Fibromyalgia (FM), one can't overlook the imperative role of sleep. Sleep dysfunctions are prevalent in CFS and FM, and understanding these disturbances is key to managing these conditions effectively. The restorative powers of sleep can make a world of difference to those battling the relentless fatigue and pain synonymous with these syndromes.

Sleep disorders in CFS and FM patients aren't just about feeling tired. There's a complex interplay between the quality of sleep and the severity of symptoms one experiences. Disrupted sleep patterns can exacerbate pain, affect cognitive function, and hinder the body's natural healing processes. It's as if your body's maintenance team is on strike, and the restoration project is indefinitely delayed.

A common complaint among CFS and FM patients is the feeling of non-refreshing sleep. You may spend hours in bed, yet wake up feeling as if you've been tossing and turning all night. This sensation of waking up exhausted, regardless of sleep duration, is a hallmark of sleep dysfunction in these conditions.

Exploring the specific types of sleep abnormalities reveals why this happens. CFS and FM sufferers often experience disturbances in their sleep architecture. The architecture refers to the structure of sleep cycles, including stages of light sleep, deep sleep, and REM sleep. It's in these deeper stages that healing and repair predominantly occur.

For instance, individuals with FM frequently have an anomaly called 'alpha-wave intrusion,' where bursts of awake-like brain activity interrupt the deep sleep stage. This intrusion can prevent sufferers from reaching the restorative stages of sleep, leading to muscle pain and stiffness upon waking.

Moreover, there's an increased prevalence of sleep disorders such as restless legs syndrome (RLS) and sleep apnea among the FM and CFS populations. These conditions not only disrupt the quantity of sleep but also severely impact its quality, leaving patients in a perpetual state of sleep deficit.

Understanding the nature of these sleep dysfunctions is a step toward regaining control over your health. Many patients aren't even aware that they have a treatable sleep disorder, attributing their tiredness solely to their primary condition. Therefore, it's essential to communicate with healthcare providers about sleep concerns.

Assessment tools, like sleep diaries and polysomnography (sleep studies), are pivotal in diagnosing and understanding the depths of sleep dysfunction. These tools can help pinpoint specific physiological changes that occur during sleep, offering insights into personalized treatment approaches.

Treating sleep dysfunctions in CFS and FM isn't one-size-fits-all. It's about finding the right combination of therapies that will work for your unique situation. Some individuals benefit from prescription sleep aids or supplements like melatonin, while others may find relief through sleep environment improvements.

Cognitive Behavioral Therapy for Insomnia (CBT-I) is another promising avenue for many patients. It deals with the psychological and behavioral aspects of sleep disturbance, helping patients develop habits and attitudes conducive to better sleep.

Pain management at night is also critical. As pain can be a significant barrier to sleep, effectively managing it with medication, relaxation techniques, or gentle exercises can aid in better slumber. Some FM patients find that a warm bath before bed or using a heated blanket can ease their muscles enough to encourage sleep.

It's worth noting that sleep medication may not be the right answer for everyone, as certain medications can actually exacerbate feelings of grogginess. Your body's response to medications is as individual as your experience with CFS or FM; what works for one person can have completely different effects on another.

Additionally, sleep hygiene practices are part of the foundation for better sleep. These involve maintaining regular sleep schedules, creating a comfortable sleep environment, and engaging in calming activities before bed. Though these might seem trivial compared to the mountain of symptoms you're facing, they're the bedrock of building healthier sleep patterns.

Lastly, let's not underestimate the power of hope and perspective. While the journey with CFS and FM can be daunting, sleep dysfunction is something that can often be improved with the right interventions. The understanding and management of your sleep issues are directly linked to your overall well-being and quality of life.

The pursuit of quality sleep is not just an act of rest; it's an active step towards reclaiming your health and vitality. Every good night's sleep is a victory, a sign that your body is healing. Embrace each restful moment, and let's continue our journey towards wellness with patience and understanding.

Strategies for Improved Sleep Hygiene and Restorative Rest

Sleep isn't just a respite from the day's demands—it's a vital player in the healing orchestra, especially for those grappling with Chronic Fatigue Syndrome (CFS) and Fibromyalgia (FM). Improving sleep hygiene and achieving restorative rest can seem like a tall order, but it's essential for the body's repair processes. With a few strategic tweaks to your routine, a blissful slumber isn't just a dream—it can be your reality.

First off, let's talk about setting the scene. Your bedroom should be a sanctuary dedicated to sleep. Consider the ambiance—the temperature, light, and noise levels. These are your sleep environment's core elements, and they need attention. Keeping the room cool, using blackout curtains to keep it dark, and minimizing noise with earplugs or a white noise machine can significantly improve your sleep quality.

What about your mattress and pillows? They should support your body, easing the pressure points typical in FM. Invest in quality bedding that makes you feel cradled and comfortable. It may seem like a luxury, but it's actually quite the necessity for restorative rest.

Establishing a regular sleep-wake schedule is crucial. Yes, your body has an internal clock, and it thrives on consistency. Aim to go to bed and wake up at the same time every day—even on weekends. This regularity strengthens your body's sleep-wake cycle, providing a sense of rhythm and making it easier to fall asleep and wake up naturally.

Banish electronics from the bedroom an hour before sleep. The blue light emitted by phones, tablets, and computers is notorious for hijacking your body's readiness for sleep by messing with melatonin production. Instead, try unwinding with a book or some gentle stretches to signal to your body that it's time to wind down.

Diet plays a role in sleep too. It's best to avoid big meals, caffeine, and alcohol close to bedtime. These can cause discomfort, keep you tossing and turning at night, or even promote visits to the restroom that disrupt your sleep.

Have you considered a pre-sleep ritual? It might include things like a warm bath, meditation, or a cup of non-caffeinated herbal tea. Such activities aren't just practices; they're signals that hug your nervous system, telling it to shift into a lower gear.

Physical activity is a great ally in improving sleep—but timing is key. Exercise can energize you, so it's best to enjoy it at least a few hours before bedtime. Gentle exercises can also help ease FM symptoms, setting the stage for a more restful night.

If your mind is a racecar zooming around at bedtime, try some relaxation techniques like deep breathing, progressive muscle relaxation, or guided imagery. These are gentle on-ramps toward the highway of sleep, guiding your mind away from the day's stress.

And let's not forget about daylight exposure. Natural light plays a vital role in regulating sleep patterns. Try to get some sunlight during the morning—this can reinforce your natural circadian rhythms, helping you feel sleepy when it's time to hit the hay.

For those moments when sleep eludes you, don't force it. Tossing and turning for hours can create an association between your bed and frustration. If you can't fall asleep within about 20 minutes, leave the bedroom and do something calming. When drowsiness taps you on the shoulder, return to bed.

Consider keeping a sleep diary. By tracking your sleep patterns and habits, you can notice what helps or hinders your sleep, and then adjust accordingly. You're gathering intel into what uniquely works for you—this can be incredibly empowering.

If a racing mind is particularly stubborn, mindfulness and meditative techniques can take the edge off. Focusing on the present moment can reduce the flurry of thoughts about the past or anxiety for the future, making space for sleep to slide into place.

There are also some natural supplements to consider, like magnesium or melatonin, that could lend a helping hand. Of course, consult with your healthcare provider first to ensure they fit neatly into your overall health plan and don't interfere with any medications you might be taking.

Lastly, be patient with yourself. Improving sleep takes time and experimentation. There's a wave of trial and error involved, but remember, each night is a new opportunity to inch closer to the rest you need and deserve. Think of this journey not as an overnight transformation but as cultivating a garden—the more love and attention you give it, the more it will flourish.

Embracing these strategies, you're not just aiming for more hours of sleep—you're reaching for a higher quality of rest. You're creating a foundation upon which healing can build, one restful night at a time.

Chapter 7:
Exercise and Movement Therapy

Navigating the delicate balance between activity and rest is essential, especially when contending with the unpredictable nature of Chronic Fatigue Syndrome (CFS) and Fibromyalgia (FM). In the context of exercise and movement therapy, this chapter delves into creating a symbiotic relationship with your body's needs, exploring how mindful, deliberate movement can foster not just physical strength but also emotional resilience. Embracing exercise isn't about pushing through pain or fatigue—it's about listening to your body and finding the sweet spot where movement becomes therapy, not a challenge. Whether it's the gentle flow of tai chi, the structured progression of a physical therapy program, or simply a walk in the fresh air, the act of moving can be transformative.

We'll uncover how individualized exercise regimes can boost energy levels, decrease pain, and improve sleep. The goal here isn't to set records or compete but to gently encourage your body to rebuild its strength and vitality at a comfortable pace. With patience and persistence, even the smallest movements can pave the way to significant improvements in your well-being, empowering you to reclaim control over your health narrative, one step at a time. So let's explore how to introduce therapeutic exercise into your life in a way that honors where you are now and where you hope to be.

The Benefits of Exercise for CFS and FM Patients

Moving your body might seem counterintuitive when you're coping with the exhausting symptoms of Chronic Fatigue Syndrome (CFS) or the pervasive pain of Fibromyalgia (FM). But embarking on a gentle journey of movement can actually be one of your staunchest allies in managing these conditions. Let's unpack the reasons why and uncover the very real rewards of incorporating exercise into your life.

Firstly, exercise—when done mindfully and at an appropriate level—has been shown to improve energy levels over time. It's a bit of a paradox; you use energy to gain more of it. However, this is the beauty of exercise. Through consistent, low-impact activity, you can gradually enhance your stamina, combatting the lethargy that often defines CFS.

For FM patients, the benefits are also significant. Regular exercise can lead to a reduction in pain and stiffness. The movement helps your muscles stay strong and flexible, preventing them from becoming tight and tender. As your strength grows, you might find that your overall pain decreases, making daily activities more manageable.

Let's not forget the mood-boosting effects of exercise. It promotes the release of endorphins, our body's natural painkillers and mood elevators. This can be incredibly beneficial, as both CFS and FM can wreak havoc on your emotional well-being.

Another advantage of exercise is improved sleep. Many CFS and FM patients struggle with sleep disturbances, but exercise can help regulate your sleep patterns. With better sleep, your body has a chance to heal and rejuvenate, which is crucial for managing these conditions.

Exercise also plays a role in managing weight. Weight control can be a challenge with CFS and FM, especially as certain medications and reduced activity levels can contribute to weight gain. Exercise helps mitigate this by burning calories and building muscle mass which, in turn, can boost metabolic rate.

Improved cardiovascular health is yet another benefit. CFS and FM can put you at a higher risk of heart disease, but regular movement helps to strengthen your heart and blood vessels, enhancing blood flow and oxygenation throughout your body.

There's also the benefit of increased self-efficacy. Successfully engaging in exercise can give you a sense of accomplishment and control over your body. This can be empowering for those who often feel at the mercy of their symptoms.

Furthermore, exercise can help with the management of other symptoms, like headaches, that can come with these syndromes. Gentle activities like yoga or tai chi can reduce tension in the muscles that contribute to headache pain.

For those dealing with the cognitive fog that often accompanies CFS and FM, movement therapy can offer some clarity. Exercise increases blood flow to the brain, which may enhance cognitive functions and help you maintain mental sharpness.

Some CFS and FM patients also experience gastrointestinal discomfort. Regular, gentle exercise helps the digestive system function more efficiently, potentially easing symptoms like bloating and constipation.

Exercise can also play a role in improving immune system regulation. While the relationship between exercise and immunity is complex, moderate activity can help reduce inflammation, which is a central feature of both CFS and FM.

Moving on a regular basis can foster a better connection with your body. You'll become more attuned to its signals and needs, which is incredibly important in conserving energy and recognizing your limits.

Of course, it's critical to approach exercise in a way that's specially tailored for CFS and FM patients. Overexertion can lead to symptom flares, so it's important to balance activity with rest. A gradual increase in activity can help mitigate the risk of post-exertional malaise (PEM).

Last but not least, exercise can be a conduit to social connections. Joining a group exercise class or walking club can provide a sense of community and support, which is valuable when you're navigating a chronic illness that can often feel isolating.

So, as daunting as it may seem, the key is to start slow, listen to your body, and recognize that movement, in its own gentle way, can be a profound part of your journey towards wellness. Each step, each stretch, each strengthening movement, is a celebration of what you can do, rather than what you can't. And that's a powerful shift in perspective for anyone on the path to managing CFS and FM.

Tailoring Activities to Individual Abilities

Balancing activity and rest is akin to finding the right melody in music—every note matters, and so does catering to your own unique rhythm. When it comes to exercise and movement therapy for those living with Chronic Fatigue Syndrome and Fibromyalgia, recognizing and honoring your current capabilities isn't just wise, it's essential. It's about discovering the movements that resonate with your body's needs, allowing for gentle progression without tipping the scales towards exhaustion. Imagine tailoring a garment to fit you perfectly; that's precisely what we aim to do with your exercise routine. By listening closely to your body's feedback and adjusting activities accordingly, you cultivate strength and stamina at a pace that won't overtax your reserves. This personalized approach ensures that each stretch, each step taken, is towards a balanced path of wellness.

Low Impact Exercises Transitioning into the realm of exercise and movement therapy, it's crucial for individuals with Chronic Fatigue Syndrome (CFS) and Fibromyalgia (FM) to focus on activities that support their healing journey without exacerbating symptoms. Gently guiding your body through low impact exercises can yield significant benefits, enhancing physical capacity and emotional well-being.

Low impact exercises are defined by their gentleness on the body, especially on the joints. They are particularly beneficial because they carry a reduced risk of injury and can be maintained over longer periods, which is essential when dealing with chronic conditions. While the idea of exercise may seem daunting, it's important to remember that even mild physical activity is better than none, particularly when tailored to your current health status.

Walking is one of the most accessible forms of low impact exercise. It's free, can be done almost anywhere, and the pace can be adjusted to match your energy levels. Even a brief walk can stimulate circulation and breathing, which in turn can help reduce pain and fatigue over time. Aim for consistency rather than distance - a daily short walk is more valuable than an occasional long one.

Swimming or water aerobics are excellent for those with CFS and FM because the buoyancy of water supports your body and reduces strain on your muscles and joints. The resistance of water provides a safe environment for building strength and endurance. Moreover, the sensory experience of being in water can be soothing for overstimulated nervous systems.

Cycling is another low impact exercise that can be adapted to suit your energy levels. Whether using a stationary bike or going for a ride outdoors, cycling helps build leg strength and cardiovascular health without putting too much pressure on the joints. Remember to start slow, listen to your body, and gradually increase the duration and intensity.

Pilates and yoga can also be modified to fit the needs of people with CFS and FM. These practices focus on core strength, flexibility, and mindful breathing. They can help manage stress, enhance posture, and decrease pain. Look for classes specifically designed for those with chronic illnesses or speak with the instructor beforehand to ensure a safe and supportive experience.

For those who find traditional exercise routines too strenuous, tai chi might be a suitable alternative. This gentle martial art focuses on slow, deliberate movements coupled with deep breathing. It's often referred to as "meditation in motion," and can be particularly beneficial for improving balance, coordination, and relaxation.

Strength training is also possible through low impact approaches. Using light weights or resistance bands, you can perform exercises that build muscle strength without overloading the system. The key is to use low weights and high repetitions, and to avoid pushing to muscle fatigue.

Since everybody is different, what works for one person may not work for another. It's crucial to customize the exercise routine to your current health status and personal preferences. The pace at which you increase activity should be gradual, and always within a range that feels comfortable and manageable for you.

Remember to warm up before beginning any exercise routine and cool down at the end; this can help prepare your body for activity and prevent post-exercise soreness. Even simple stretches or light movements can serve as an adequate warm-up for low impact exercises.

It's also worth noting the importance of consistency over intensity. It may be tempting to push yourself on days when you feel more energetic, but doing too much could lead to a setback. It's better to engage in a moderate amount of activity regularly rather than occasional bursts that may trigger symptoms.

The benefits of incorporating low impact exercises into your routine extend beyond physical health. Regular physical activity can also lead to improved sleep, reduced anxiety, and even a brighter mood. As you nurture your body with gentle movement, you may find a sense of empowerment and control in your journey with CFS and FM.

When integrating low impact exercises into your life, it's key to work in partnership with a healthcare professional who understands your condition. They can help you create a balanced exercise plan that aligns with your therapeutic goals and current level of health.

In addition, keeping a journal can be an invaluable tool in documenting your exercise routine, tracking progress, and evaluating how different types of activities affect your symptoms. Over time, this record can help you and your healthcare team fine-tune your approach to exercise.

Lastly, be patient and compassionate with yourself. Celebrate every achievement, no matter how small it may seem. Each step taken in the direction of wellness, each gentle stretch, each breath during a meditative exercise, is a testament to your strength and determination to live well with CFS and FM.

Stretching and Strengthening Routines

For individuals coping with Chronic Fatigue Syndrome (CFS) and Fibromyalgia (FM) should be approached with care and compassion. Living with these conditions means finding a balance between rest and activity, listening intently to what the body needs, and gradually introducing exercise to avoid excessive fatigue or a flare-up of symptoms.

Let's start with stretching, which is an essential component of any physical activity plan. Stretching can aid in increasing flexibility, reducing stiffness, and even alleviating pain. For someone with CFS or

FM, the goal is to stretch gently and consistently. Think of the body as tight elastic that needs slow and careful pulling to become more pliable; rushing or pushing too hard can snap it back to square one.

A routine might begin with simple neck rolls, easing into each position and holding it for a few breaths. Progress might feel slow, but remember that every small movement is a victory. Gradually, the routine can incorporate shoulder stretches, arm reaches, and wrist rotations, all done while seated or lying down to conserve energy.

The lower body also benefits from a good stretch. Ankle circles can promote blood flow, especially for those who may experience numbness or tingling in their extremities. Gentle leg raises and knee-to-chest stretches can relieve some of the tension that builds up from periods of inactivity. As flexibility increases, yoga poses like the "Cat-Cow" can introduce a broader range of motion, altogether enhancing the suppleness of the spine and torso.

When it comes to strengthening, it's crucial to start with the core muscles — the torso's stabilizers. Weak core muscles can lead to poor posture and increased pain. Pilates exercises, modified as needed, can be incredibly effective. The "Pelvic Tilt" and "Dead Bug" exercise are two examples that strengthen the core without requiring a lot of energy. Breathing deeply during each exercise helps oxygenate the body and ensures that the muscles are being nourished.

Building strength in the arms and legs can follow, using resistance bands or light weights. Bicep curls and wrist curls, when done slowly and with lower repetitions, can build arm strength without causing undue strain. Similarly, seated leg presses and side leg lifts can strengthen the lower body, possibly improving balance and stability.

Consistency is key. Establishing a daily routine, even if it's just for a few minutes, can contribute to a sense of routine and well-being. On days when energy is particularly scarce, the routine can be shortened or modified. It's not about pushing through pain or exhaustion; it's about maintaining movement in whatever way feels manageable.

It's also important to note the mind-body connection during these exercises. Visualization techniques can be useful, such as picturing the muscles lengthening and strengthening as each exercise is performed. This can make the routine more than just a physical practice; it becomes a time for mental rejuvenation and connection as well.

Another component of these routines is hydration and proper nutrition. Ensuring that the body is well-hydrated and that you are consuming foods that support muscle health — such as those rich in protein, magnesium, and omega-3 fatty acids — can complement the physical efforts being made.

Some might find it helpful to track progress, jotting down which exercises were done, the number of repetitions, and any changes in how they feel. Others might prefer to stay in the moment, focusing on the experience instead of the outcome. Both approaches are valid, and it really comes down to what motivates and encourages each individual.

Remember, with conditions like CFS and FM, a gentle push is sometimes necessary but a hard shove is never recommended. Recovery and strengthening take time and patience. Celebrate small wins — each stretch, each strengthening move is a step towards better health and improved energy levels.

For times when movements are limited due to flare-ups or fatigue, even simple breathing exercises can maintain a connection to the routines. Diaphragmatic breathing, practiced while seated or lying down, can help maintain core strength and provide a sense of calm.

Community support can also play a role. Joining a group, whether online or in person, where others understand the highs and lows of these routines can be incredibly validating. Sharing what works, what doesn't, and learning from each other's experiences can foster a sense of camaraderie and community, which is beneficial for mental and physical health.

Lastly, it's crucial to incorporate days of rest into any stretching and strengthening routine. Rest days allow the body to recover and help prevent the "boom and bust" cycle where overexertion leads to prolonged periods of inactivity. It's about finding that sweet spot where movement and rest coexist harmoniously, enabling you to take care of your body without exhaustion or pain.

Remember to honor your body's limits, embrace your abilities, and keep faith in the possibility of improvement. A stretching and strengthening routine tailored for CFS and FM isn't just about the physical benefits; it's about reclaiming a sense of agency over your body and a commitment to gently nudging its boundaries. It's about resilience in motion, one stretch, one strength move, one breath at a time.

Chapter 8:
Cognitive Behavioral Therapy and Mindfulness

Emerging from the previous discussions on the tangible aspects of managing Chronic Fatigue Syndrome (CFS) and Fibromyalgia (FM), we pivot to the profound influence of the mind in Chapter 8. Cognitive Behavioral Therapy (CBT) presents as a beacon of hope, shifting perspectives and sharpening tools to navigate the fraught seas of chronic illness. It's less about changing circumstances, which often remain stubbornly consistent, and more about adjusting sails—the thoughts and beliefs that can make winds either threatening gales or guiding breezes. Pairing neatly with CBT, mindfulness offers a different kind of sanctuary—a return to the present moment where pain and fatigue don't eclipse the entirety of one's existence, but simply exist as transient experiences among many. The emphasis here isn't on the broad-strokes solutions, but on individual empowerment, on cultivating a mental landscape where acceptance cradles ambition, and where each breath can be a step towards reclaiming command over a seemingly relentless tide.

Enhancing Mental Health Through CBT

Continuing our exploration of paths to wellness, let's turn our focus to the transformative potential of Cognitive Behavioral Therapy, often abbreviated as CBT. CBT is a therapeutic approach that has shown significant promise for those grappling with Chronic Fatigue Syndrome (CFS) and Fibromyalgia (FM). It operates on the concept that our thoughts, emotions, and behaviors are interconnected and that altering one of these components can instigate change in the others.

CBT begins with the premise that maladaptive thinking patterns contribute to the persistence of distressing symptoms. For instance, someone with FM might believe 'I'll never be able to have an active life again,' which can lead to feelings of hopelessness and a decrease in attempts to engage in activity. Recognizing these thought patterns is pivotal. Once identified, CBT works to challenge and modify these beliefs, promoting a more balanced and positive mindset.

At its core, CBT is about empowerment. The therapy equips you with a set of tools to take control of the 'mental chatter' that so often exacerbates our physical experience of pain and fatigue. It's not unusual to feel stuck in a loop of negative self-talk and prophesying the worst. CBT nudges you to question the validity of these thoughts and to reframe them into ones that serve you better.

Engagement with CBT also introduces the concept of behavioral activation. When living with CFS and FM, you might understandably reduce your level of activity to avoid pain and fatigue. However, this can lead to a cycle of inactivity that exacerbates symptoms further. CBT encourages gradual increases in activity, structured in a manageable way to help break this cycle.

To complement behavioral activation, CBT promotes practical problem-solving strategies to manage daily tasks. Let's say you're dreading a trip to the grocery store. CBT would have you break down the task into smaller steps, assess each step for potential challenges, and then plan accordingly. Perhaps you decide to write a list, shop during off-peak hours, or use an online delivery service. Tackling challenges in bite-sized chunks can make them feel less overwhelming.

Another CBT strategy is to develop a better awareness of personal limits and to respect those boundaries. For many, overexertion on 'good days' leads to crash-and-burn cycles. CBT helps in recognizing your baseline of activity, which can be crucial in managing your condition effectively.

The importance of stress reduction in managing CFS and FM cannot be overstated, and CBT offers numerous techniques to manage stress. Deep breathing exercises, progressive muscle relaxation, and guided imagery can act as a switch to calm the nervous system. Lower stress levels have a direct impact on the intensity of symptoms experienced.

Self-monitoring is an invaluable CBT technique. By keeping a journal of your thoughts, feelings, and symptoms, you can start to uncover patterns. Perhaps you'll notice that certain thoughts precede a flare-up of symptoms or come to understand how your mood affects your pain levels. This self-awareness can be transformative.

CBT is not just a solo journey; it's about connectivity. It encourages the active involvement of families and friends. Learning effective communication skills can help others understand what support you need and when you might need space. It's about building a team around you that can support your CBT journey.

An essential ingredient of CBT is setting achievable goals. Small, incremental goals provide a roadmap to recovery, giving you a sense of accomplishment and a forward trajectory. For someone with CFS or FM, something as seemingly simple as a daily walk around the block can be a significant victory.

It's essential to recognize that CBT doesn't claim to be a cure for CFS or FM. Instead, it's a method of improving quality of life by coping better with symptoms. By helping you change how you think about your condition, it can lead to changes in how you feel and behave, which can make an enormous difference in your daily life.

Whilst CBT is predominantly delivered by a trained therapist, the principles can be implemented individually, offering flexibility for those who might have mobility or energy limitations. There are online CBT resources, books, and even apps that can guide you through the process from the comfort of your home.

Likewise, let's not overlook the group-based CBT interventions. They offer a sense of community and understanding that's deeply comforting. Sharing struggles and victories with peers can foster a deep sense of solidarity and can be particularly impactful for those feeling isolated by their chronic conditions.

Integrating CBT into your wellness routine can be pivotal. But it requires an open mind, dedication, and patience. Change won't happen overnight, but small and consistent efforts can yield meaningful progress in how you manage CFS and FM.

Remember, despite the challenging days, healing and improvement are possible. Embracing CBT principles can be a powerful step towards not just enduring these conditions but living a fuller, more satisfying life in spite of them. So, take it one day at a time, and let cognitive behavioral therapy gently guide you towards your personal wellness horizon.

Incorporating Mindfulness and Stress Reduction Practices

Mindfulness and stress reduction practices are essential components to managing the complexities of life with chronic fatigue syndrome (CFS) and fibromyalgia (FM). If you're grappling with the incessant noise of pain and fatigue, you might find incredible relief in the quietude of mindfulness. It's more than a practice; it's a nurturing way of life that invites calm into your world.

Throughout this chapter, we will explore different facets of mindfulness and how they can be seamlessly woven into your daily routine. Remember, these aren't quick fixes but rather gentle, ongoing practices that can shift your response to stress and potentially alleviate some CFS and FM symptoms.

Starting with the basics—mindfulness is the art of being present. It's about noticing your thoughts, feelings, sensations, and the environment around you, without judgement. For those with CFS and FM, this can be particularly powerful. Pain and fatigue often demand attention, but mindfulness teaches you to observe them without letting them dominate your experience.

One of the core practices of mindfulness is meditation. It's a tool that sharpens your focus and brings clarity to the mind. Even a few minutes each day can make a difference. Begin by finding a comfortable spot and focusing on your breath. As thoughts or pains arise, acknowledge them, and gently guide your attention back to your breathing.

Breathing exercises are also central to stress reduction. Deep, diaphragmatic breathing can calm the nervous system and promote relaxation—a boon for anyone with CFS and FM. Try inhaling deeply through your nose, holding for a couple of seconds, and then exhaling slowly through your mouth. This simple practice can be your haven in moments of distress.

Body scan meditation is another beneficial practice. It involves mentally scanning your body for areas of tension and consciously releasing it. Start from your toes and move upward, taking note of each body part. Where you find tension, breathe into it, and on the exhale, imagine it flowing away. This not only promotes relaxation but also increases body awareness.

Progressive muscle relaxation (PMR) is a related technique that involves tensing and then relaxing different muscle groups. It's especially useful if you're experiencing muscle pain or stiffness from FM. By alternately tensing and relaxing, you teach your body the difference between the two states, which can reduce overall muscle tension.

Mindfulness isn't just for quiet, solitary moments. It can be integrated into everyday activities like eating, walking, or even while doing chores. When eating, for instance, savor each bite, pay attention to the textures and flavors, and notice the sensations of fullness. This can transform a routine activity into a rich, grounding experience.

Guided imagery is a wonderful tool as well. It's a form of focused relaxation that helps create harmony between the body and the mind. By visualizing calming images or scenarios, your body responds as though what you're imagining is real, bringing about a sense of peace and reducing stress hormones in the body.

Yoga and tai chi blend physical movement with mindfulness, proving to be excellent for both body and mind. These gentle exercises can help stretch and strengthen muscles, improve balance, and reduce stress. While engaging in these movements, focus on your breath and the sensations in your body to foster a meditative state.

Gratitude journaling can be a profoundly uplifting practice. Start or end your day by writing down things you're grateful for. They don't have to be grand; even small pleasures can make a significant impact. This practice trains the brain to seek out the positive, creating a buffer against the challenges posed by CFS and FM.

Mindful communication is also key. When talking with others, listen fully, speak authentically, and remain present. This not only enriches your interactions but also helps mitigate the misunderstandings that often accompany chronic illness. It builds a bridge of empathy and connection, which is so vital when feeling isolated by your condition.

Lastly, don't underestimate the power of nature in promoting mindfulness. Spending time in green spaces can have a soothing effect on the mind and body. Whether it's a walk in the park, gardening, or simply sitting by a window with a view of trees, connecting with nature can be an invigorating stress reducer.

Mindfulness and stress reduction shouldn't be seen as another task on your to-do list; rather, they're a refuge. Like a soft, warm blanket on a chilly day, these practices are there to comfort and support you. They're a testament to the strength within you—the strength to face each moment with grace and composure.

In this journey with CFS and FM, it's vital to embrace a compassionate approach toward yourself. Incorporating mindfulness and stress reduction practices offers a way to not just cope, but to thrive amidst the challenges. By anchoring in the present, you ground yourself in a state of being that is both resilient and serene.

Chapter 9:
Alternative and Complementary Therapies

In our ongoing exploration of living well with Chronic Fatigue Syndrome (CFS) and Fibromyalgia (FM), we now venture into the world of *alternative and complementary therapies*, an inviting realm that offers a rich tapestry of options beyond conventional medicine. This chapter is dedicated to those who are curious about integrating additional modalities into their healing regimen to potentially ease symptoms and enhance quality of life. We'll look at the mosaic of treatments available—like acupuncture, which may reduce pain and restore energy flow, or massage therapy, a hands-on approach that can alleviate the deep muscular discomfort that so often shadows FM. We'll also touch upon chiropractic care, a practice that might realign and relieve, while refraining from delving into details on herbs and supplements, as each therapy is a stepping-stone on the distinct path you carve for your wellness journey. With an open mind and cautious optimism, let's embrace these therapies as possible allies, remembering that each person's response is as unique as their fingerprint.

Exploring Acupuncture, Massage, and Chiropractic Care

In our quest for wellness, particularly when dealing with the tangle of symptoms in Chronic Fatigue Syndrome (CFS) and Fibromyalgia (FM), many of us look beyond conventional medicine. We're often seeking relief that taps into the body's innate healing mechanisms. That's where alternative therapies such as acupuncture, massage, and chiropractic care come into play. These practices offer diverse ways to address pain and enhance well-being, and they have garnered both anecdotal and research-supported acclaim.

Acupuncture, with its roots in traditional Chinese medicine, aims to restore balance and promote healing by stimulating specific points on the body. It's thought to tweak the body's energy flow or Qi (chee), and for some with CFS and FM, this stimulation can translate into reduced pain and improved energy. Imagine fine needles creating tiny sensations, prompting your body to redirect its attention and resources to areas that need healing.

From the acupuncturist's table, let's shift to massage therapy, a treatment that kneads away the layers of tension that CFS and FM patients often carry. Not only does massage provide a soothing escape from discomfort, but it also fosters better circulation, reduces muscle stiffness, and can improve sleep — something chronic illness warriors deeply value. The touch of a skilled therapist can be both healing and validating, acknowledging the physical effects of these often invisible illnesses.

Chiropractic care, too, holds a unique place in our holistic toolkit. This discipline focuses on the body's structure, principally the spine, and its function. Chiropractors employ adjustments to align the body properly, which in turn can alleviate pain, improve movement, and boost overall health. For those grappling with the joint discomfort and postural pain of CFS and FM, chiropractic interventions can sometimes be like a reset button, bringing a sense of alignment and ease.

Understandably, there's often skepticism before embarking on these therapies. How can needles, human touch, or spinal adjustments help conditions as complex as CFS and FM? The evidence is complementary, and while not a panacea, these therapies can be integrated components of a broader management plan. They might not be the magic cure, but the therapeutic benefits for some can feel pretty magical.

Of course, every body is a universe unto itself, and what works for one person may not work for another. This is why it's essential to approach acupuncture, massage, and chiropractic care with cautious optimism. Start with a certified practitioner who has experience with CFS and FM — their expertise can be invaluable in navigating the nuances of these conditions.

Getting the most out of these therapies also involves careful timing and pacing. For those with limited energy reserves, it's vital to schedule appointments at times when the body is most receptive, considering the possibility of post-treatment fatigue. It's a delicate dance — listening deeply to your body's signals and responding with grace. Be patient with yourself as you explore the potential of these therapies.

When trying acupuncture, it's common to have a course of several treatments to judge its effectiveness. In each session, you might discover that your body responds unexpectedly, with relief felt in areas that weren't even on your radar. The power of targeted relief can shine a light on the complex interplay of symptoms you're experiencing.

With massage therapy, the relationship with your therapist is key; it's a partnership, where communication about pressure, areas of focus, and your comfort level is crucial. The therapist's hands become conduits of healing energy, easing not just the physical pain but also soothing the emotional stress that often accompanies chronic illness.

And within the domain of chiropractic care, it's common to have a phased approach. Initial visits may focus on immediate pain relief, followed by corrective care, and finally, maintenance to prevent future issues. The chiropractor's adjustments aim to restore your body's alignment, which can be pivotal to managing CFS and FM symptoms.

Sharing your experiences with these therapies among support groups and with your healthcare team can help you gauge your progress. It also contributes to the broader conversation about what works in the management of these complex conditions. You become a storyteller, sharing invaluable insights that can light the way for others on a similar path.

It's important to monitor how your body reacts to these treatments. While many find relief, some may experience exacerbation of symptoms or new discomforts. Always listen to what your body is telling you and maintain an open dialogue with your practitioners. They should be partners in your journey to wellness, making adjustments to their approaches as needed.

While contemplating these therapies, don't discount the emotional and psychological benefits. The act of being cared for, of being seen and touched, can have deeply therapeutic effects on the psyche. The acknowledgment of your pain and the concerted efforts of a professional working to alleviate it can be profoundly affirming.

Insurance coverage for these therapies can sometimes be tricky. It's worth researching what your plan includes and advocating for yourself if necessary. Resources are out there to help make these treatments more accessible, from sliding scale fees to community clinics.

In the world of CFS and FM, where conventional medicine sometimes falls short, these alternative modalities offer rays of hope. Tap into these ancient and enduring forms of healing and discover how they might harmonize with your body's unique rhythm. Perhaps acupuncture, massage, or chiropractic care can become a treasured note in the symphony of your treatment — playing a part in a more profound and tuneful experience of health and vitality.

Ultimately, your wellness journey is your own. It's a path paved with discoveries and choices that resonate with your individual needs and aspirations. So, keep an open mind and heart as you explore the potential of acupuncture, massage, and chiropractic care. They offer gateways to relief and empowerment, letting you tune into a fuller sense of well-being — a harmony of body, mind, and spirit that every person deserves to experience.

The Use of Herbs and Alternative Supplements

Embarking on a journey of managing chronic conditions like Chronic Fatigue Syndrome (CFS) and Fibromyalgia (FM) often requires us to look beyond conventional medicine. Within that search, many find solace in the ancient wisdom and emerging science behind the use of herbs and alternative supplements. While the path to wellness isn't one-size-fits-all, incorporating natural remedies may serve as another beacon of hope for those navigating these complex illnesses.

Herbal therapies have been used for millennia to treat a myriad of ailments. With an increasing number of individuals with CFS and FM looking for holistic treatment options, it's important to dive into how such supplements can potentially aid in symptom management. It's critical to understand that while these therapies can complement traditional treatments, they should never completely replace the advice and care of your healthcare provider.

Among the herbal supplements gaining attention, adaptogens such as Ashwagandha and Rhodiola have shown potential in supporting the body's ability to cope with stress – a common trigger for CFS and FM flare-ups. These powerful herbs may help modulate the stress response system within your body, offering a more balanced approach to fighting fatigue and enhancing mental clarity.

Another common symptom for CFS and FM patients is pain, and this is where herbs like turmeric, which contains the active compound curcumin, may play a role. Turmeric is highly regarded for its anti-inflammatory properties and when used in moderation, might contribute to reducing joint and muscle pain associated with inflammatory responses in the body.

When fatigue wears you down, it can be tempting to turn to stimulating herbs. However, it's wise to proceed with caution. Substances like guarana and high concentrations of ginseng, which can be potent energy boosters, must be used judiciously as they may exacerbate anxiety or disrupt sleep patterns in sensitive individuals.

Speaking of sleep, valerian root and lemon balm are commonly heralded for their sedative properties. When sleep eludes you, they may aid in calming the mind and promoting a more restful state, though it's always pivotal to ensure they don't interact negatively with any medications you might be taking.

A mentally and physically weary spirit can often find a gentle lift from St. John's Wort, used for centuries as a mood enhancer. While this herb shows promise for those with mild depression symptoms, it's imperative to recognize its potential interactions with other drugs and to consult your healthcare professional before use.

Muscle spasms can be a distressing part of FM, and herbs like cramp bark and magnesium-rich supplements could offer muscle relaxation. These natural relaxants are known for easing muscle tension and soothing tightness without the harsh side effects sometimes associated with prescription muscle relaxants.

Additionally, digestive issues often accompany FM and CFS, and herbs like peppermint and ginger are celebrated for their gut-soothing characteristics. Whether through teas or capsules, these herbs can alleviate nausea and improve digestive function, contributing to overall comfort and well-being.

While herbs and supplements show promise, they're not without potential risks. It's crucial to be discerning, looking for quality and purity in products. The supplement market is largely unregulated, so do your homework, seek recommendations from trusted sources, and keep your healthcare provider in the loop.

Dosage and consistency are two sides of the same coin when it comes to the effectiveness of herbal remedies. Developing a routine under the guidance of a knowledgeable professional could make the difference in whether you see tangible benefits from these natural products.

Not all experiences with herbs and supplements are created equal, and what aids one person's recovery may not have the same effect for another. It's important to listen to your body and monitor for any adverse reactions, adjusting your regimen as necessary.

One can't ignore the potential interactions between herbs and pharmaceutical medications. Always discuss new supplements with your pharmacist or doctor to ensure that they won't interfere with your current treatments or cause harmful side effects.

Lastly, it's worth considering the role of lifestyle alongside natural supplementation. A holistic approach that combines diet, exercise, sleep hygiene, and stress management provides a solid foundation that may be further strengthened with the considered use of herbs and alternative supplements. Optimizing your overall health strategy can help keep both mind and body in the game.

Herbs and alternative supplements could provide pieces to the complex puzzle of managing CFS and FM. With the right approach and professional guidance, they may enhance your journey towards better health and a richer, more vibrant life amidst the challenges of chronic illness.

Chapter 10:
Navigating Relationships and Social Dynamics

As we continue piecing together the mosaic of wellness, it's crucial to consider the intricate web of relationships and social interactions that define our lives. For those grappling with the invisible burdens of Chronic Fatigue Syndrome and Fibromyalgia, the terrain of interpersonal connections can be as challenging as managing symptoms. In this journey, the art of communication is your compass, guiding you to articulate your needs, set boundaries, and foster understanding with those who matter most. Crafting robust support systems isn't just beneficial; it's vital. This chapter empowers you to bridge the gaps between your experiences and the perceptions of others, fortifying the bonds that construct your personal community. It's about embracing vulnerability, enlisting allies in your health odyssey, and cultivating a nurturing environment that resonates with empathy and solidarity. Remember, you're not navigating these waters solo; with every shared story and extended hand, your network becomes a vessel of hope and collective strength, sailing towards a horizon of mutual support and deeper connection.

Communication Strategies with Family and Friends

Navigating the tides of chronic illness isn't a journey one should ever have to take alone. The impact of Chronic Fatigue Syndrome (CFS) and Fibromyalgia (FM) extends beyond the physical; they touch every aspect of a person's life, including relationships with family and friends. Developing clear and effective communication strategies is essential in ensuring that the support systems surrounding individuals with these conditions are both sturdy and nurturing.

First and foremost, it's critical to be open about your diagnosis. This isn't always easy. There's often a nagging fear of misunderstanding or disbelief given the invisible nature of CFS and FM symptoms. However, sharing your experience provides a foundation for empathy and support. When you tell your loved ones what you're going through, use simple but descriptive language, and don't shy away from expressing your feelings and limitations.

Educating your inner circle is an extension of openness. Arm them with knowledge about CFS and FM. They may not fully grasp the science, but understanding the basics can help them make sense of your experience. Share literature, invite them to attend doctor's appointments, or find support groups where they can learn from the experiences of others.

Clear communication also involves setting boundaries. It's easy to overextend to avoid letting others down, but this can exacerbate your condition. Be honest about what you can and can't do. Let your loved ones know this isn't about your desire to spend time with them but about managing your health.

Conversely, it's essential to express what kind of support you need. People often want to help but may not know how. Do you need someone to just listen, help with chores, or accompany you to medical appointments? Being specific can channel their desire to help in the most beneficial way.

There may also be times you'll need to communicate during a flare-up or a particularly bad day. Establish a signal or phrase that lets your family and friends know you're struggling and need space or assistance.

This pre-agreed upon shortcut can alleviate the stress of having to explain your situation when you're feeling at your worst.

It's important to recognize the power of gratitude in these relationships as well. Always take a moment to acknowledge the effort and support your loved ones provide. This not only strengthens your bond but can make them feel appreciated and seen.

Remember, however, that communication involves listening as well. Encourage your family and friends to share their feelings about your illness. It affects them, too, and acknowledging their emotions and struggles builds mutual understanding.

Be prepared for setbacks and misunderstandings. Patience is key. Sometimes it takes multiple conversations for people to get a sense of what you're dealing with. If a family member or friend reacts negatively or expresses disbelief, give them time. They may need to process the information in their own time.

Having a plan for social interactions can also help. Prioritize activities and rest so you can enjoy the time with friends and family. If you're attending an event, have an exit strategy in case you become overwhelmed or too fatigued.

Pivot communication to suit your energy levels. Perhaps a text message or email might suffice when a phone call feels too taxing. Let people know that your response time may vary depending on how you feel, and that short replies don't mean you value their messages any less.

Involve your loved ones in your wellness journey. Celebrate small victories together and include them in the creation of self-care plans. This can help them feel involved and gives them tangible ways to support you.

Importantly, seek professional guidance if communication barriers persist. Therapists and counselors trained in chronic illness dynamics can provide valuable tools and mediation that can help clarify, heal, and strengthen the lines of communication.

Don't forget to nurture relationships outside of the context of your illness. Make sure to engage in discussions and activities that aren't centered around your condition. This helps maintain the balance and richness of your relationships, reminding everyone involved that your illness doesn't define you.

Lastly, practice empathy for yourself and for others. Balancing the social dynamics of chronic illness is not without its challenges. Compassion, both for your situation and for the learning curve others are on, can smoothen the rough edges that come with navigating this complex territory. With empathy, patience, and clear communication, the bonds with your family and friends can transform into one of your greatest sources of strength on this journey.

At the end of the day, communication is about connection. It's about weaving the threads of understanding, support, and love through the fabric of your relationships to create a safety net that holds you steady on your path to wellness. Even on the toughest days, knowing that your voice has been heard and your experience validated can be the beacon that guides you through the fog of chronic illness.

Building Support Systems and Community Connections

As you navigate the complexities of chronic conditions like Chronic Fatigue Syndrome (CFS) and Fibromyalgia (FM), fostering a robust support system and culling meaningful community connections can significantly buoy your spirits and bolster your resilience. It's not just about seeking solace; it's about forging partnerships that empower and elevate your wellbeing.

Firstly, let's discuss the importance of recognizing your personal network. Your support system may encompass family, friends, colleagues, or members of support groups who understand the ebbs and flows of living with a chronic illness. It's invaluable to surround yourself with those who get it—empathy is a balm for the weary soul. Honesty with these individuals about your condition and its limitations can foster a deeper understanding and more meaningful support.

Building bridges with others who share similar experiences can mitigate feelings of isolation. Joining support groups, whether in person or online, provides a platform to exchange stories, strategies, and sometimes just to vent. Shared experiences are powerful; they validate your struggles and victories alike. Many communities are home to CFS and FM support groups where you can form these essential connections.

Volunteering, as health permits, can also be a lifeline to the world beyond your illness. Whatever your interests or abilities, there's likely a volunteer opportunity that's a great fit. This can provide a sense of purpose and community involvement that may be missing when health issues overshadow other aspects of life.

Consider the role of local establishments like libraries, community centers, or places of worship. These venues often host events, classes, or groups that can be gentle on your body while offering social stimulation. Tai chi, gentle yoga, or book clubs can introduce you into the local fabric without overwhelming your system.

Furthermore, hobbies and interests shouldn't fall by the wayside. Whether it's crafting, gardening, or music, these activities can be therapeutic and a means to meet others with similar interests. They can be adapted to suit your energy levels on any given day. Explore local clubs or online communities centered around your hobbies.

When you're up for more social interaction, hosting small get-togethers or participating in low-energy meetups are good options.

These can be casual coffee dates, potluck dinners where everyone contributes a dish (saving you energy), or just a cozy afternoon with close friends. The key is to keep it manageable and stress-free.

Technology can be a powerful ally in building community connections. Social media groups and forums specific to CFS and FM patients allow you to be part of a community from the comfort of your home. Though it's essential to be mindful of the time spent on devices as it can sometimes lead to fatigue.

Education can be a form of support too. Enlightening those around you about CFS and FM can deepen their understanding and patience with your condition. This might involve sharing articles, books, or even inviting them to attend a support group meeting or medical appointment with you.

It can't be overstressed how vital it is to cultivate self-compassion. Recognize your worth outside your illness and strive to nurture connections that reinforce this. Your life is multifaceted, and while CFS and FM are a part of it, they don't define your entire being.

It's also crucial to acknowledge that some days will be tougher than others in terms of socializing. Listen to your body; it's okay to cancel plans if you need to rest. A true support system understands the unpredictability of your circumstances.

For caregivers and family members, it's important to build your own support systems as well. Caregiver support groups, both in person and online, can provide a space for sharing experiences and techniques that can help manage the emotional and physical demands of caregiving.

Lastly, remember that building and maintaining a support system is an ongoing process. People might come and go, but each connection has the potential to add value to your life. Stay open to new relationships and nurture the ones that nourish you. Real connection, empathy, and support don't go unnoticed and can indeed make the road less daunting.

Embark on this journey of connection with your whole heart. While it might require some energy and vulnerability, the benefits of a warmth-filled community—a collection of hearts that understand and support you—are immeasurable. With every step you take toward building this network, you're crafting a firmer foundation for your daily life, strengthening you for the path ahead.

In conclusion, your social landscape doesn't have to be vast to be valuable. It's about quality, not quantity. So tend to it with the same care you would a garden, and watch as it blooms, providing a vibrant backdrop to your life, even on days when CFS and FM seem to cast a long shadow.

Chapter 11:
Working with Healthcare Professionals

In navigating the complexities of Chronic Fatigue Syndrome (CFS) and Fibromyalgia (FM), building a strong alliance with healthcare professionals is not just beneficial—it's critical. Embarking on this journey begins with a proactive mindset towards your medical care, recognizing that a collaborative and informed relationship with doctors, specialists, and therapists is the cornerstone of effective management. It's about choosing a healthcare team that is not only knowledgeable about CFS and FM but also one that aligns with your personal health philosophy and understands the uniqueness of your situation. Advocacy plays a key role here, as you'll need to be your own voice in medical settings; confidently expressing your concerns, asking the hard questions, and seeking clarifications to make informed decisions about your treatment plan. Remember, it's a partnership where your input is invaluable and when both sides work together, the path towards wellness becomes clearer and more attainable. You're an integral part of this team, and finding healthcare professionals who respect and support your contribution can truly make a world of difference in your healthcare experience and outcomes.

Choosing Your Healthcare Team

Embarking on a journey towards health and wellness with chronic conditions like Chronic Fatigue Syndrome (CFS) and Fibromyalgia (FM) requires assembling a team of healthcare professionals who not only understand these complex syndromes but also respect and support your unique circumstances. Building this team is no minor task, and it begs careful consideration, as each member plays a vital role in devising and implementing your treatment plan.

Your healthcare team might consist of a variety of professionals, from primary care physicians and rheumatologists to physical therapists and mental health counselors. Each practitioner brings a specialized set of skills and knowledge to your care. Therefore, it's crucial to choose individuals who are not just experts in their fields but are also empathetic and open to a multidisciplinary approach.

Primary care physicians often serve as the central pivot for your healthcare team. They are typically the first contact for managing your overall health and coordinating with other specialists when necessary. Look for a doctor who is not only adept at general healthcare but is also knowledgeable about CFS and FM—or at least willing to learn and listen to your experiences.

Rheumatologists can be pivotal in the treatment of FM, given that they specialize in musculoskeletal and autoimmune conditions. Their expertise in managing pain and understanding the nuances of FM is invaluable. When choosing a rheumatologist, consider their familiarity with FM and their willingness to work in tandem with other professionals on your healthcare team.

For CFS, a specialist with a background in infectious diseases or neurology may offer the most insight. These professionals can help unravel the complexities of CFS, addressing the neurological and potential infectious components of the condition. Their specialized knowledge can be particularly enlightening when conventional approaches yield limited progress.

Given the impact CFS and FM can have on your mental well-being, including a mental health professional on your team is beneficial. Whether it's a psychologist, psychiatrist, or counselor, make sure they're sensitive to the psychological toll of living with chronic illness and can provide robust support, including techniques for managing stress, depression, and anxiety that commonly accompany these conditions.

Physical therapists (PTs) trained in managing chronic pain conditions can offer tailored movement therapies to help maintain muscle function and reduce discomfort. They understand the balance between activity and rest and can guide you in establishing a routine that aligns with your energy levels. Selecting a PT familiar with the limitations imposed by CFS and FM is critical for a program that supports recovery instead of exacerbating symptoms.

If you're exploring complementary treatments, such as massage therapy, acupuncture, or chiropractic care, consider practitioners who have experience with CFS and FM patients. This ensures they understand how to modify treatments to accommodate for sensitivities and for potential flare-ups these conditions may entail.

Likewise, given the importance of nutrition in managing CFS and FM, a dietician or nutritionist can be an integral part of your healthcare team. Choose a professional who can provide personalized dietary advice that is responsive to your body's needs and is aware of any food sensitivities or digestive issues that often accompany these conditions.

Building this diverse team might feel daunting, especially when energy is a limited resource. Starting with one trusted healthcare provider can be a solid first step. This can be a physician or a nurse practitioner whom you trust and who appreciates the complexities of your condition. This individual can help you navigate and expand your team based on your evolving needs.

It's also essential to recognize that finding the right healthcare professionals may require some trial and error. Just as every patient's experience with CFS and FM is unique, so too is each healthcare professional's approach to treating it. Be patient and give yourself permission to change team members if the fit just isn't right.

When choosing your healthcare team, don't underestimate the value of communication. You'll want professionals who not only speak to you with clarity and compassion but also listen intently and validate your experiences. Shared decision-making should be at the heart of your interactions, with a focus on respectful partnership rather than a top-down directive.

Lastly, remember that you are the most critical member of your healthcare team. Your insights into your own body and your lived experience are invaluable data points in managing your condition. An effective team not only acknowledges this but actively encourages your input and participation in every aspect of your care plan.

Finding and choosing a healthcare team is a significant step in managing CFS and FM. It's a dynamic process that values expertise, empathy, and patient empowerment. With the right team in place, you can more confidently manage your symptoms and work towards your wellness goals, even in the face of the unpredictability these conditions often present.

In summary, prioritize professionals who are not only technically adept but who also show a genuine commitment to working collaboratively with you on your health journey. With these collaborative relationships in place, healing and improved quality of life are within reach, despite the challenges that CFS and FM pose.

Advocacy and Self-Representation in Medical Settings

Navigating the healthcare system can be like trying to solve a complex puzzle, especially when you're living with conditions like Chronic Fatigue Syndrome (CFS) and Fibromyalgia (FM). Being your own advocate and effectively representing yourself are indispensable skills that will help ensure your healthcare experience is as beneficial as possible. It's about communicating your needs, making informed decisions, and steering your treatment in a direction that aligns with your personal health goals.

Healthcare advocacy starts with understanding your condition. While previous chapters delved into the science and personal stories behind CFS and FM, this knowledge base becomes your power in a medical setting. If you understand your symptoms and how they affect you, you can better articulate these experiences to your healthcare providers. Remember, you're the expert on your own body and experiences. Your insights into how your symptoms manifest and fluctuate are vital pieces of information for anyone involved in your treatment.

Equipped with knowledge, it's crucial to communicate effectively. Clear, concise communication can bridge the gap between patient and provider. When preparing for an appointment, try writing down your main concerns and what you hope to get out of the meeting. This preparation can help keep the conversation focused and productive. Have a list of questions and don't hesitate to ask for clarifications. Misunderstandings can lead to inappropriate care, so it's better to over-communicate than under.

In advocating for yourself, you must also know your rights as a patient. These include the right to privacy, informed consent, and the right to make decisions about your own care. If a proposed treatment doesn't sit right with you, it's your prerogative to discuss alternatives. You're not just a passive recipient of healthcare; you're an active participant. By knowing your rights, you empower yourself to engage in your care plan more assertively and responsibly.

A key part of self-representation is building a rapport with your healthcare team. When your providers see you as a person, not just a patient, they're more likely to listen and take your concerns seriously. Share your struggles and victories, big and small, with your healthcare team. Establishing this connection can transform your healthcare experience from impersonal to collaborative.

Documentation is another cornerstone of effective self-advocacy. Keep thorough records of your appointments, symptoms, treatments, and any side effects. This not only helps you track your progress but also provides your healthcare team with vital information that can influence your care. When your symptoms and experiences are documented, they're harder to dismiss or overlook.

Even with preparation, communication can sometimes break down, and you may feel like you're not being heard. In such situations, it's important to remain calm and assertive. Use "I" statements to express how you feel about the care you're receiving and what you need from your healthcare provider. This non-confrontational approach can reopen lines of communication and help you get back on track.

When it comes to treatments and interventions, be curious and do your homework. Investigate new therapies, but maintain a healthy skepticism. Just because something is touted as a "miracle cure" does not mean it is effective or safe for everyone. Discuss these treatments with your healthcare team and consider their advice carefully. Your providers can help you weigh the potential benefits against the risks and costs.

It's also critical to be realistic about the limitations of the healthcare system. Providers are often pressed for time and resources, which can lead to shorter appointments and longer wait times. Use your time wisely and understand that your healthcare provider's short responses aren't necessarily a sign of disinterest, but perhaps a reflection of systemic pressures.

Don't forget, if you're having trouble advocating for yourself, it's okay to bring in backup. A trusted friend or family member can accompany you to appointments for support. They can also help advocate on your behalf, take notes, and ask questions that you might not think of in the moment. This support can ease the stress of self-advocacy and ensure that all bases are covered during your visit.

Treat each healthcare encounter as a learning experience. Reflect on what went well, what could have gone better, and how you might approach things differently next time. This reflection can lead to continued improvement in how you represent and advocate for yourself in these situations.

In some cases, you may feel that a provider isn't a good fit for you. Listen to your gut. It's okay to seek a second opinion or to look for another provider altogether. Your well-being is paramount, and it's important to work with healthcare professionals who understand, respect, and effectively respond to your needs.

Lastly, involve yourself in patient communities. Connecting with others who have CFS and FM can provide not only emotional support but also practical advice on navigating the healthcare system. These communities often share tips on effective self-advocacy and may recommend healthcare professionals known to be sympathetic and knowledgeable about your conditions.

Remember, your journey to wellness is unique, and self-advocacy is an ongoing process. As you continue to engage with healthcare professionals, your skills in self-representation will grow stronger. Each step you take as your own best advocate brings you closer to the personalized care you deserve and moves you along the path to managing your health in a way that fits your life.

Celebrate every success in your advocacy efforts, no matter how small they may seem. Each victory is another stride in your journey toward empowerment and better health. With tenacity and perseverance, you can shape the narrative of your healthcare experience to one of collaboration, understanding, and mutual respect.

Chapter 12:
Planning for the Future

When dealing with chronic conditions like Chronic Fatigue Syndrome and Fibromyalgia, it's natural to yearn for a roadmap that charts out a less daunting journey. That's why this chapter—dedicated to plotting a course into your future—is a beacon of empowerment. Getting a grip on your narrative means crafting goals that aren't just wishful thinking, but blueprints for the life you long to lead. It invites you to strike a delicate balance between aspiration and the contours of reality, ensuring dreams aren't castles made of sand, but fortresses built to endure. It's about tailoring your environment to your unique needs, ensuring your living space and workplace are not just zones you endure, but sanctuaries where wellness and productivity are in a harmonious dance. Consider this chapter a compass to guide you through the murky waters of uncertainty, an ally to help you visualize and forge a future that aligns with your deepest longings while standing firm in the truth of today.

Setting Realistic Goals and Expectations

When dealing with chronic conditions like Chronic Fatigue Syndrome (CFS) and Fibromyalgia (FM), it can feel like you're navigating through a perpetual fog, uncertain of when it will lift. However, setting realistic goals and expectations is a beacon that can guide you through the haze, illuminating your path forward. These goals serve not just as milestones but also as powerful mechanisms for tracking progress, maintaining motivation, and enhancing your sense of control over your life.

As you chart your course, remember that every journey begins with a single step. Your goals should be attainable and measurable. Setting superhuman expectations will only lead to disappointment and discourage your progression. Start small, perhaps with daily tasks that support your overall health management, like a mindful breathing exercise or a nourishing meal. Small victories create positive feedback loops that can empower you to take the next step.

It's essential to recognize that living with CFS and FM often means adapting to a fluctuating symptom landscape. This can mean that what you're capable of on one day might differ from the next. Flexibility is your ally in this journey. Define your goals with the built-in understanding that adjustments may be necessary, and that's perfectly okay. It's not stepping back; it's smart strategizing.

Your expectations of yourself should be compassionate and patient-centric. It might be tempting to push through on a good day, but understanding your boundaries is critical. Pacing is a term you'll hear often, representing the delicate balance between activity and rest. Listen to your body—it will tell you when it's time to slow down.

Building a solid support network—including healthcare providers, family, friends, and support groups—is an essential part of setting realistic goals. Share your aspirations with this trusted circle; they can offer perspective, help you stay on track, and provide support when you hit inevitable bumps in the road.

Creating a visual representation of your goals can be incredibly helpful. It might take the form of a chart, a journal, or even a vision board. This gives you a tangible reminder of what you're working towards and makes the process of achieving goals more engaging and less abstract.

Now, beyond the day-to-day, setting long-term goals is equally important. While achieving them might take longer or require more flexibility, these goals give you something to aspire to over time. Maybe it's a particular hobby you want to engage in again or a trip you would like to take. Ensure these larger goals are broken down into smaller, more manageable steps to sidestep feeling overwhelmed.

Being realistic also means accepting that progress is not always linear. You will face good days and difficult ones, and that's part of the natural ebb and flow with CFS and FM. Acknowledge and celebrate your good days, and be kind to yourself on the tougher ones. Progress isn't about never falling; it's about learning how to get back up, no matter how many tries it takes.

Don't overlook the goal of rest. In a society that glorifies busyness, honoring the necessity of rest can feel counterintuitive, but rest is productive for individuals with CFS and FM. It can be as necessary as any other treatment or management strategy. Make rest a goal, not an afterthought.

When setting personal development goals, remember that your mental and emotional health are as important as physical health. Objectives might include practicing daily gratitude, engaging in CBT or mindfulness, or spending time in nature. These contribute significantly to your overall well-being.

For those navigating work while managing CFS and FM, recognizing your value extends beyond physical capabilities. Setting goals around work might involve exploring flexible work arrangements, learning new skills for a more suitable role, or advocating for workplace accommodations that address your unique needs.

Lastly, it's crucial to review your goals regularly. As your condition changes, so too will your capabilities and priorities. Regularly reassessing your goals ensures they remain relevant and supportive rather than becoming an outdated source of stress. Celebrate the progress you've made, and adjust as needed to keep your aims in harmony with your current situation.

Throughout this journey, remember that goals can evolve. Just as a river carves its path through a landscape, so too will your experience with CFS and FM shape your goals. Embrace the process of adaptation and recognize the strength in being malleable. Your ability to reshape expectations, to bend without breaking, is a testament to your resilience.

In conclusion, when setting realistic goals and expectations, be your own best advocate and gentlest critic. With each step forward, you solidify your path toward wellness. Use your goals as guideposts and allow them to light your way through the dimmer moments. With thoughtful planning and compassionate self-awareness, your future becomes a landscape of potential—ready to be mapped out, step by step.

With these thoughts in hand, dream bravely, plan carefully, and walk forward with confidence. Your future is not just something to be reached but shaped by your actions and perspectives. And in doing so, you will find not just progress, but moments of joy and triumph along the way.

Adaptations and Accessibility: Home, Work, and Beyond

When we talk about living with Chronic Fatigue Syndrome (CFS) or Fibromyalgia (FM), it's no secret that the path to wellness isn't just about medical treatment—it's also about shaping your environment to support your health. Adapting your home, work, and other areas of life can be transformative and this section aims to ignite your imagination with practical advice on forging a life that meets you where you are.

At home, think comfort and functionality. Investing in ergonomic furniture that supports your posture can alleviate pressure points and reduce pain. Functional adaptations may include voice-activated home systems that can control lights, temperature, and electronics without you needing to move. Small changes, like reorganizing your kitchen to put frequently used items at arm-level, can conserve energy and reduce strain.

Don't overlook the bathroom, an oft-used space that can be a true friend or foe. Consider a shower chair and non-slip mats to mitigate fatigue and prevent falls. Grip bars and an elevated toilet seat can also make a significant difference in maneuvering safely and maintaining independence.

Work is another critical topic. The Americans with Disabilities Act gives you the right to request reasonable accommodations from your employer. This might include flexible working hours, working from home options, or specialized equipment. Talk openly with your employer about your needs. Remember, they can't help if they don't understand your daily battles. Use your voice as an advocate for your well-being.

Think about your technology too. There are myriad software and apps designed to help people with chronic illnesses. From note-taking applications that decrease the need to type to speech-to-text software that eases communication, tech has your back.

Mobility aids might be a subject to consider as well. If walking long distances is a challenge, using a cane, walker, or even a mobility scooter can offer newfound freedom. It's not about labeling yourself as disabled; it's about embracing tools that can propel you towards more vivacity and joy in your day-to-day life.

Organization is your silent partner in this journey. Keeping your home and workspaces clutter-free minimizes the energy required for routine tasks. Designate specific places for your essentials, and you'll reduce the stress of searching when brain fog descends.

Let's remember that rest is not idleness. Creating quiet, restful spaces within your home can serve as safe havens for your body to recuperate. Serene colors, soft lighting, and comfortable bedding can all contribute to a restorative environment.

When thinking further afield, consider your transportation needs. Being a passenger rather than a driver on longer journeys can be less tiring, and planning for rest breaks can help manage your energy levels. In many areas, disability placards or plates can grant you closer parking spots, which can be a considerable relief on difficult days.

Let's be honest, this isn't a journey you can make without the support of your nearest and dearest. Enlist the help of family and friends to make your living space more accessible. Even something as simple as opening jars or changing lightbulbs can become shared tasks to conserve your energy for more meaningful activities.

It can be intimidating to reimagine your life with CFS or FM, but small, consistent changes can create a profound impact over time. The goal is not just to make accommodations—it's to create a life that feels full, productive, and happy within the parameters of your condition.

Financial considerations are undoubtedly part of the puzzle. Investigate grants, financial aid, or community resources that can help fund home modifications or mobility aids. Some organizations are dedicated to supporting individuals with chronic illnesses, and reaching out to them could open the door to helpful resources.

Finally, remember to maintain flexibility in your approach. What works today may not serve you tomorrow, and that's okay. Your needs will evolve as you navigate CFS or FM and so too should your environment. Be willing to reassess and adapt as needed to continue supporting your wellness journey.

Take each step towards adaptation and accessibility as an act of self-care. You're crafting a world in which you can thrive, not just survive. Your home and work can become sanctuaries that foster healing and productivity.

In closing, while many parts of living with CFS or FM can feel overwhelming, taking control where you can is empowering. Design your personal and professional life to accommodate your needs, leaning on the tools and strategies available. Every effort to create an accessible environment is an investment in your future—a future brimming with hope and potential.

Chapter 13:
Embracing a Hopeful Horizon

As we near the close of our journey through the realms of Chronic Fatigue Syndrome (CFS) and Fibromyalgia (FM), it's important to pause and reflect on the paths we've traversed and the vistas that lie ahead. We've delved deep into the science and stories, unraveled the mysteries of pain and fatigue, and charted courses through the complexities of diet, sleep, and therapy. Now, we stand at a vantage point, looking out upon a hopeful horizon.

The challenges that come with CFS and FM can often feel like impenetrable fog, shrouding life's joys and obscuring the way forward. Yet, with each step we take, empowered by knowledge and support, the fog begins to lift, revealing the infinite potential for healing and growth. You're not alone on this trek, and the strides made by so many before us have illuminated a trail bristling with promise.

Nutrition has served as a fundamental cornerstone, offering sustenance and strength to bodies wearied by CFS and FM. Ingesting the right blend of nutrients and adhering to dietary strategies tailored to personal needs doesn't just fuel the body; it kindles the spirit, imbuing each day with the possibility of better health and vitality.

Managing pain and fatigue is, without question, a daily ordeal, but it's one that's evolved with our deepening understanding. From pharmaceutical remedies to holistic therapies, the tools at our disposal are diverse and ever-improving. Employing these assets creatively and judiciously can help reclaim command over one's life.

Don't underestimate the transformative power of restorative sleep. Its role in healing is indisputable and cultivating practices to achieve restful nights is a triumph worth every effort. Sleep is not just a pause from daily struggles; it's a rejuvenating balm, mending the weary fibers of our beings.

Exercise and movement, once perhaps thought of as adversaries, have become allies in managing CFS and FM. Adopting tailored activities that respect our bodies' limits lets us greet the day with renewed strength and guards against the stagnation that can come with chronic illness.

Wrapped in the soothing embrace of mindfulness, cognitive behavioral therapy emerges as a beacon of mental resilience. It's a sail to catch the winds of change, steering us away from the turbulent waters of anxiety and depression, and guiding us towards serene shores.

With the exploration of alternative therapies, we've opened doors to new sanctuaries of healing. Whether it's the precise touch of acupuncture, the therapeutic strokes of massage, or the ancient wisdom of herbs, these complementary practices enfold us in a tapestry of diverse healing threads.

The strength of our personal relationships has been both tested and fortified. Communication, ever so crucial, became a bridge over tumultuous waters, connecting us with those who may not fully grasp our experiences but stand ready to offer support. Building a supportive community is like weaving a net that catches us when we fall and lifts us when we're ready to rise.

Working in tandem with healthcare professionals, we've honed the art of advocacy and self-representation. It's a dance, sometimes graceful, sometimes challenging, but always pushing towards collaboration that is respectful, empathetic, and constructive.

Planning for the future isn't just about setting goals; it's about adapting to the ever-changing contours of life. We learn to construct our environments, activities, and aspirations not merely to accommodate but to enrich, making them accessible bastions from which we can engage with the world meaningfully and joyously.

This horizon before us radiates with the light of countless individuals—each battling their struggles, each contributing to a collective wellspring of knowledge and compassion. The horizon holds an invitation to not just survive, but to thrive; to not merely exist, but to live with a fullness that defies the limitations of CFS and FM.

Remember, the horizon is not a fixed line where the earth meets the sky. Rather, it's a symbol of possibility, always moving, always expanding as we journey forward. Embrace this horizon with open arms and an open heart, carrying with you the wisdom and experiences shared through these pages.

As this chapter concludes, your personal narrative goes on, each day writing a line, each action painting a stroke of your masterpiece. Embrace every sunrise as an opportunity, each challenge as a lesson, and every moment of joy as a treasure.

May you venture forth with a spirit of adventure, a heart full of courage, and a resolve that's unshakeable. Onwards towards that hopeful horizon, where tomorrow awaits with the promise of peace, well-being, and the sweetest victories, both big and small.

Appendix

As we tie the loose ends of our discussions on Chronic Fatigue Syndrome and Fibromyalgia, it's important to equip you with extra tools and resources to support your journey. This Appendix is that toolbox—a collection of materials and tidbits promising to assist you in the daily management of these complex conditions. Here, you'll stumble upon a curated assemblage of practical items such as checklists, charts, and perhaps a recipe or two that didn't find a home in previous chapters but are too valuable to overlook.

The road towards wellness isn't a predictable one; it can zig and zag in ways you never foresaw. That's why it's crucial to have a reservoir of resources at your disposal—consider them your personal aids on this path. These additional pieces of information are meant to complement the text, giving you a broader base of knowledge and strategies to pull from. When you're grappling with a particularly tough day, glance through these pages. They might harbor the exact advice or encouragement you need to push through.

Within these final pages, soak up the distilled wisdom that can act as a soothing balm to your fatigue-taxed mind or a gentle push when you're navigating a pain flare-up. Let them serve as a guidepost to understanding your body's unique language and needs. Embrace the comfort that comes from knowing that, even when the book ends, your support system can still expand, transforming each page of the Appendix into a steppingstone towards reaching your personal, brighter horizon.

And remember, while the journey to wellness is as personal as it gets, you don't have to walk it alone. You've likely gathered a wealth of knowledge and insights from the previous chapters. Now, with this Appendix, you're further adding to your mental library an array of supplementary materials that reinforce that expertise, making the management of your condition that much more attainable.

Dive into these extra resources with the knowledge that they're crafted to assist you in fine-tuning the balance in your life, creating a harmony between rest and activity, providing nutritional support, enriching your mental wellbeing, and ensuring you're well-equipped to articulate your needs to those around you. As you navigate these final pages, let them be a gentle reminder that your story continues and every day holds the potential for improved health and happiness.

Glossary of Terms

Embarking on your wellness journey, you may encounter an array of terms that can sometimes feel overwhelming. This glossary is meticulously crafted to help you understand the key concepts related to Chronic Fatigue Syndrome (CFS) and Fibromyalgia (FM) as you read through this book. It's tailored to support patients, caregivers, healthcare professionals, researchers, and anyone interested in learning about these conditions and their management.

A

Acupuncture: A traditional Chinese medical practice using fine needles to stimulate specific points on the body, aimed at restoring balance and reducing pain.

Advocacy: The act of supporting or speaking out for oneself or others, especially in the context of healthcare and patients' rights.

Anti-inflammatory Diet: A way of eating that aims to reduce inflammation in the body, which can be particularly beneficial for those dealing with CFS and FM.

C

Chiropractic Care: A form of alternative therapy that involves the manipulation of the spine and other parts of the body to alleviate pain and improve function.

Cognitive Behavioral Therapy (CBT): A type of psychotherapy that helps individuals change unhelpful patterns of thinking and behavior to improve emotional regulation and develop personal coping strategies.

Chronic Fatigue Syndrome (CFS): A complex, long-term illness characterized by extreme fatigue and other symptoms not explained by an underlying medical condition.

E

Energy Conservation: Techniques and strategies used to manage fatigue by pacing activities and protecting energy reserves.

Exercise Therapy: A regimen or treatment plan involving physical activity designed to strengthen the body and improve health outcomes for those with CFS and FM.

F

Fibromyalgia (FM): A chronic disorder known for widespread musculoskeletal pain, fatigue, sleep issues, and memory and mood problems.

H

Herbs and Alternative Supplements: Natural products used to provide relief from symptoms associated with CFS and FM, often emphasizing holistic approaches to health.

I

Inflammation: The body's immune response to injury, infection, or irritation, which can contribute to the symptoms experienced by patients with CFS and FM.

M

Mindfulness: The practice of maintaining a moment-by-moment awareness of thoughts, feelings, bodily sensations, and surrounding environment with openness and acceptance.

Massage Therapy: The manipulation of soft tissues in the body to alleviate pain and promote relaxation and healing.

N

Non-Pharmaceutical Therapies: Treatment options that don't involve medication, such as physical therapy, mindfulness, and dietary changes.

P

Pacing Techniques: Approaches for managing and adjusting one's activity level to avoid exacerbating CFS and FM symptoms.

Probiotics: Beneficial bacteria that are consumed through certain foods or supplements to help maintain or restore healthy gut flora.

R

Restorative Rest: Quality sleep that enables physical and mental recovery, particularly important for those with CFS and FM.

S

Sleep Hygiene: The practices, habits, and environmental factors that are conducive to sleeping well on a regular basis.

Supplements: Products taken orally that can contain a variety of nutrients, such as vitamins, minerals, enzymes, or herbs, intended to add nutritional value to the diet.

As you continue to flip through the pages of this guide, use this glossary to empower your understanding. Remember, you're not just absorbing information; you're equipping yourself with the tools to stride more confidently on your path to wellness. And remember, you're not alone on this path.

Resource Guide for Patients and Caregivers

Navigating the landscape of Chronic Fatigue Syndrome (CFS) and Fibromyalgia (FM) can often feel like traversing an intricate maze without a map. That's why understanding the resources available to you is like discovering a compass in your pocket. This guide is designed to provide direction and support, unveiling a collection of tools for patients and caregivers that serve as beacons of hope and empowerment.

Living with a chronic ailment can sometimes feel isolating, but it's important to remind yourself that you're not alone. Support groups, both local and online, offer a sanctuary where you can share experiences, advice, and encouragement. They're a place where understanding meets empathy, and where silence is often filled with nods of acknowledgment. Within these circles, you'll find stories of resilience that fuel your own determination.

Equally vital is the role of proper healthcare providers, but finding the right team can seem daunting. Look for practitioners who not only specialize in CFS and FM but also respect your experiences. Patient advocacy organizations often provide directories of healthcare professionals versed in these conditions, which can be a good starting point to finding the help you need.

Information is power, so staying informed on the latest research and treatment approaches is crucial. Websites of reputable medical institutions, research papers, and journals specializing in CFS and FM are valuable reserves of knowledge. However, be cautious and critically evaluate your sources to avoid misinformation.

Another cornerstone of managing CFS and FM is nutrition. While this resource guide won't delve into specifics—since they are covered extensively in other chapters—know that there are dietitians and nutritionists who understand the unique needs of those living with chronic illnesses. Seeking their expertise can make significant strides in your path to wellness.

Don't underestimate the power of counseling and therapy, which can help alleviate the mental and emotional burdens that often accompany CFS and FM. Therapists who specialize in chronic illness can provide coping strategies and cognitive-behavioral techniques that empower you to navigate the psychological complexities of your condition.

When it comes to pain management, a variety of professionals, from pain specialists to physical therapists, stand ready to design a tailored approach for you. Remember, every person's experience with pain is unique, so open communication about what works and what doesn't is key to getting the most appropriate support.

Pacing and energy management classes or workshops can be incredibly advantageous. Occupational therapists, often found through local hospitals or clinics, can teach you how to balance activity with rest, conserving your energy for the things that matter most.

Sleep specialists are another resource that can't be overlooked. Their guidance on improving sleep hygiene can directly impact your quality of life, offering techniques to secure the restorative rest your body craves.

Exploring complementary and alternative medicine opens new avenues for relief and healing. Acupuncture, massage therapy, and yoga practitioners often work with those affected by chronic pain conditions, and some have additional training and focus on CFS and FM.

Bolstering your social networks reinforces that support is not limited to medical professionals. Friends, family, and community organizations can be invaluable, offering assistance from running errands to providing a listening ear. Community centers and churches often have programs or know individuals willing to help those with chronic health challenges.

Furthermore, vocational counselors could significantly benefit those striving to maintain or re-enter the workforce. They can advise on workplace accommodations, disability benefits, or career transitions that better suit your health needs.

Educational materials like books, pamphlets, and educational DVDs available in health libraries and online platforms can enrich your understanding of CFS and FM, supplementing the knowledge gained in various chapters of this book.

Remember, while the journey through CFS and FM is intensely personal, it does not have to be a solitary one. Fabricate your patchwork of support by weaving together medical resources, personal connections, and the timeless wisdom of those who walked this path before you. Be gentle with yourself as you traverse this intricate landscape, buoyed by the support and guidance that surrounds you.

Lastly, embrace technology in your journey. Apps that track symptoms, offer meditation or mindfulness exercises, and manage medication schedules can play a supporting role in your day-to-day management of CFS and FM.

As you continue flipping through the pages of this guide, let optimism be your steady companion. The coupled synergy of knowledge and support not only lightens the load but also makes the path ahead more navigable. Take it one step at a time, armed with the right resources and an unwavering commitment to your wellness journey.

Research and Study Summaries

As you've journeyed through the chapters of this book, you've absorbed a great deal of information about Chronic Fatigue Syndrome (CFS) and Fibromyalgia (FM), from symptoms to management strategies. But what anchors our understanding and continuously propels it forward are the diligent efforts of researchers who strive to unravel the complexities of these conditions. In the Research and Study Summaries section, we will highlight significant studies that have shed light on CFS and FM, providing you with insights that not only inform but also inspire.

The study of CFS and FM is a dynamic field, with new discoveries emerging regularly. What's fascinating is seeing how recent research dovetails with personal experiences, validating what many patients have known intuitively about their own bodies. For instance, studies examining the impact of nutrition on symptom management align with the advice given in Chapter 4, advocating for an anti-inflammatory diet to help ease symptoms.

Complex studies investigating the biological underpinnings of CFS and FM, discussed in Chapter 2, have unearthed evidence that there's much more to these conditions than we once thought. Scientists are delving into genetic factors, immune system dysfunctions, and even the role of microbiome diversity in these illnesses, providing a more comprehensive picture of their nature and how they can be approached therapeutically.

In understanding the role of pain and its management, we can look to research highlighted in the summaries that explores various pharmaceutical options and non-pharmaceutical therapies, identifying promising treatments and also considerations and potential side-effects for those living with CFS and FM. This parallels the discussion on pain management strategies covered in Chapter 5.

Research into sleep dysfunctions is particularly poignant for those wrestling with the disruptive rest patterns often associated with CFS and FM. Studies have demonstrated the importance of sleep quality over quantity, and our summaries will point to the research that aligns with the approaches and strategies observed in Chapter 6.

Exercise, though a challenging prospect for many dealing with CFS and FM, has been repeatedly shown to offer benefits. Research summarized in this section dovetails with Chapter 7's focus on movement therapy, illustrating how carefully tailored activities can make a significant positive impact on individuals' health.

Within the field of mental health, cognitive behavioral therapy (CBT) and mindfulness practices stand out as particularly effective tools for managing the psychological impact of CFS and FM, as underscored in Chapter 8. Our summaries will reflect recent studies that validate these approaches, offering encouragement to those for whom these strategies have been life-changing.

Turning towards alternative and complementary therapies, such as acupuncture, massage, and chiropractic care—topics deeply explored in Chapter 9—research summaries provide evidence that underscores the potential value and benefits of integrating these treatments into one's wellness routine.

Patient and healthcare provider relationships are pivotal to successfully navigating CFS and FM. Summaries of studies on effective communication and self-advocacy, as well as choosing the right healthcare team that Chapter 11 dedicates its focus to, are crucial in offering evidence-based strategies that empower patients.

Building upon the importance of social relationships and support systems discussed in Chapter 10, summaries of sociological studies bring to light how crucial these factors are in managing CFS and FM. The research emphasizes the need for understanding and supportive networks that can dramatically influence the well-being of an individual.

Looking to the future, as Chapter 12 suggests, it's essential to have goals and expectations grounded in reality. The studies we summarize present findings about the trajectory of CFS and FM, providing valuable foresight for patients, caregivers, and healthcare professionals alike.

Moreover, research into workplace and home adaptations demonstrates how adjustments in one's environment can mitigate the impact of CFS and FM. This insight ties back to the discussions about planning for the future and ensuring accessibility in all facets of life.

The ongoing study of CFS and FM is rich with promise and potential. Each study summarized represents a piece of the puzzle, bringing us closer to understanding these complex conditions. As new treatments are trialed and lifestyle modifications are tested, the research community's contributions are invaluable to providing hope and practical pathways for improved quality of life.

Finally, as we compile these summaries, we remain committed to offering updates in a field that is ever-evolving. Just as the management and treatment of CFS and FM are personalized, so too is the research diverse and tailored to various aspects of these conditions. These studies are more than just data; they symbolize the ongoing quest for knowledge and progress, illuminating the path toward wellness and resilience.

May this collection of research and study summaries serve as a source of knowledge, hope, and inspiration, affirming that you're not alone on this journey. Each finding reinforces the global dedication to better understanding CFS and FM, bringing us all one step closer to a future where managing these conditions becomes a story not solely of survival, but of thriving.

www.ingramcontent.com/pod-product-compliance
Lightning Source LLC
Chambersburg PA
CBHW051447280526
45785CB00003B/1461